A FISTFUL OF VITAMINS
> gulped before breakfast . . . are you protecting your health or fooling yourself?

"RUSSIAN PENICILLIN"
> —can garlic really lower blood pressure?

YOU CAN LOSE MORE THAN WEIGHT
> when you diet, if you don't compensate for the nutrients you're missing.

IS THERE AN ALMOST "PERFECT" FOOD?
> Yes—and it's probably not what you think it is.

The host of vitamins, minerals and food supplements and the claims made for them make nutrition a tangled and confusing jungle for most of us. Now Earl Mindell, acclaimed nutritional expert, has written this basic, easy-to-follow guide, which will allow each reader to choose his or her own path to improved health through informed nutrition, with full understanding of his or her own special requirements and how to meet them.

Other books by Earl L. Mindell, R.Ph., Ph.D.
Earl Mindell's Vitamin Bible
Earl Mindell's Vitamin Bible for Your Kids

Earl Mindell's

QUICK & EASY Guide to Better Health

Keats Publishing, Inc. ⚕ New Canaan, Connecticut

THE INFORMATION IN THIS BOOK IS NOT IN-
TENDED AS MEDICAL ADVICE, ONLY AS A GUIDE
IN WORKING WITH YOUR DOCTOR.

**EARL MINDELL'S QUICK & EASY GUIDE TO
BETTER HEALTH**

Pivot Health Edition, 1982

Copyright © 1978, 1982 by Earl Mindell, R.Ph., Ph.D.

ISBN: 0-87983-271-1
Library of Congress Catalog Card Number: 82-80701

Printed in the United States of America

PIVOT HEALTH BOOKS are published by
Keats Publishing, Inc.
27 Pine Street, Box 876
New Canaan, Connecticut 06840

This book is dedicated to...
Alanna, Evan, Alice, Noah, Joseph
THE FUTURE

I wish to express my thanks to the following people whose help and encouragement are greatly appreciated:

Gail Mindell, Bernard Bubman, R.Ph., Jane Hamilton, Tonya Shreeve, Annette Bennett, Marsha Tokareff and Mel Rich, R.Ph.

EARL L. MINDELL, R.Ph., Ph.D.

What They Mean

USRDA	United States Recommended Daily Allowance
IU	International Units
USP	United States Pharmacopoeia Units
RE	Retinol Equivalents

Table of Contents ─────────────

Foreword _____

Why another book on nutrition, you might ask?

Well, I felt that a book was needed to answer a few questions that were left unanswered by my colleagues in other books. First, why you should take supplements, and second, just as important, how and when you should take your supplements.

I have endeavored to bring the most up-to-date research into this book. Whenever possible, there will be reference guides listed for further study.

Nutrition is a fascinating field which never ceases to amaze me. Come along with me through the following pages and find out what foods you should increase your intake of and which ones you should avoid.

SOME IMPORTANT DATES
IN THE HISTORY OF NUTRITION

1869	DNA (deoxyribonucleic acid) discovered by Miescher.
1897–1906	Eijkman proved that beriberi was a dietary deficiency and that a component of rice polishings (B1) could cure it.
1911	Casimir Funk isolated crystals with B-complex activity. He coined the name vitamin from the Latin "vita"—life plus amine.
1913	Michaelis and Menten isolated chlorophyll.
1917	McCollum showed that xerophthalmia (night blindness) is due to lack of vitamin A.
1922	McCollum showed that lack of vitamin D causes rickets.
1922	Vitamin E was isolated at the University of California, and called the antisterility factor.
1924	Vitamin E given its name.
1926	Sumner isolated an enzyme and proved it to be a protein.
1928–1932	Szent-Györgyi isolated vitamin C.
1930–1933	Northrop isolated crystalline pepsin and trypsin.
1932	Warburg discovered vitamin B2 or riboflavin.

1936	Vitamin E was renamed tocopherol, when it was isolated from wheat germ oil
	From the Greek:
	  "Taco"—childbirth
	  "Phero"—bring forth

1938	Williams discovered pantothenic acid.
1938	Stevens isolated vitamin B6 (pyridoxine).
1951	Krebs isolated B15 (pangamate).
1958	Krebs patented vitamin B17 (amygdalin).

THE PRESENT

These vitamins are known today; more have yet to be discovered.

A; B-complex group: B1 (thiamin), B2 (riboflavin), B3 (niacin, niacinamide), B5 (pantothenic acid), B6 (pyridoxine), B10, B11 (growth factors), B12, B13 (orotic acid), B15 (pangamic acid), B17 (amygdalin); paba; choline; inositol; C,D,E,F (fatty acids); G (riboflavin); H (biotin); K,L (necessary for lactation); M (folic acid); P (bioflavonoids); T (growth-promoting substances); U (extracted from cabbage juice).

Supplements——
Why, when, how and which_____

Why take vitamins?

It is of the utmost importance for you to understand the role of vitamins in our life sustenance. If you were to ask a random sampling of people why they take vitamins, you would probably hear something like this:

"I take vitamins because I need them."

"I take vitamins because everyone I know takes them."

"If there's something in it for me, I want it."

"I take vitamins because my wife makes me."

"My doctor told me to take them."

"I had an ailment and found improvement after taking vitamins."

1

"I read a book on nutrition by Adelle Davis and she recommended taking vitamins."

"I saw a doctor on television who advocated them."

Vitamins occur in all organic material. Some organic matter contains more of one vitamin than another, and in greater or lesser amounts. Therefore you might say, if I eat the "right" foods or a well-balanced diet, I will get all the vitamins I need. You are right. However, very few of us do eat this mythical diet. Most of the foods we eat have been processed, for example bread or cereals. The foods in the marketplace today are depleted in nutrients. The term "enriched" is seen everywhere. This means that almost all the vitamins and minerals have been extracted and a few synthetic nutrients have been added to keep the government happy.

When and how to take vitamins

Since vitamins are foods, hence the synonym "food supplement," they are best absorbed when taken with other foods and minerals. So the best time to take them is after meals, and as evenly throughout the day as possible.

Since the water-soluble vitamins, especially B-complex and vitamin C can be excreted in the urine, a regimen of after breakfast, after lunch and after dinner gives you the highest body level. If this is not convenient, then half the amount taken during the day should be after breakfast and half after dinner. If you must take your vitamins all at one time, then taking them after the largest meal of the day will usually give the best results. Thus, after dinner, not after breakfast, is the most desirable time.

Minerals and vitamins are mutually dependent on each other for proper absorption. Vitamin C aids in the absorption of iron. Calcium aids in the absorption of vitamin D and zinc aids in the absorption of vitamin A. So take minerals and vitamins together.

The human body operates on a twenty-four hour cycle. Your cells do not go to sleep when you do, nor can they exist without continuous oxygen and nutrients. Therefore, for best results with vitamins, space them out as evenly as possible during the day.

How long do vitamins last?

Vitamins should be stored in a cool, dark place away from direct sunlight in a well-closed container. They do not have to be stored in the refrigerator unless you live in a desert climate.

Vitamins should be guarded from excessive moisture. When you open your container, place a few kernels of rice at the bottom of the bottle. Rice works as a natural absorber of moisture.

If vitamins are kept cool and away from light in a well-sealed container, they should last for two to three years. Once a bottle is opened, you can expect twelve months of shelf life.

Today all labels should have an expiration date. If the bottle you are buying does not have one, buy another brand.

Why are time release vitamins better?

The B-complex and C vitamins are water soluble. They cannot be stored in the body as fat soluble vitamins can. Therefore, they are quickly absorbed into the bloodstream and rapidly, within two to three hours, are excreted in the urine, no matter how large the dose may have been.

Time release vitamins are made by a process in which vitamins are enrobed in their own micro-pellets or tiny time pills. They are then combined into a special base for their release in a pattern that assures absorption over six to twelve hours. This gradual absorption permits the tissues greater utilization of the vitamins.

Why take chelated minerals? What are they?

Chelation is the process by which mineral substances are combined with amino acids and are changed into their digestible form. Common mineral supplements such as bone meal and dolomite are not chelated and must first be acted upon in the digestive process to form chelates before they are useful to the body.

Chelated supplements are made by the same process nature uses to chelate minerals in the body. Many people cannot perform the chelating process efficiently in their bodies; therefore, many of the mineral supplements they take are of little use.

Are minerals as important as vitamins?

Yes! The body can synthesize some vitamins but it

cannot manufacture a single mineral. Yet minerals are biological activators necessary to the body. For example, magnesium is involved in 78 percent of our known enzyme systems.

What destroys vitamins?

We have been told about over-processed food. The chemicals which bleach and change and "preserve" foods destroy vitamins and minerals. Some of them are put back in "enriched" food, but not all of them. Many drugs deplete the body's reserve of vitamins (See pp. 107–113). Pollution in the environment is certainly another vitamin-destroying factor.

Random vitamin notes:

According to the most recent information, 20 to 50 percent of Americans do not meet the U.S.R.D.A. (Recommended Daily Allowance) for at least one or more of the vitamins:

> A
> C
> B1 (thiamin)
> B2 (riboflavin)
> Folic acid

Dieters or meal skippers usually eliminate foods that contain many vitamins, including C, E and B complex. Sickness, including fevers and colds, can lower the level of vitamins in your blood. Senior citizens, who have difficulty chewing and digesting their food often have poor eating habits. This condition can lead to an insufficiency of water-soluble vitamins, including B complex and C; and long-term antibiotic users can be depleted in vitamin B complex.

The vitamins and minerals _____

Here is a vitamin-mineral list for quick reference
to the natural sources of the vitamins and minerals:
what they do in the body and their deficiency signs.
The deficiency symptoms described in these pages
could occur only when the daily intake of the vitamins has been less than the minimum requirement over a prolonged period. These non-specific
symptoms do not alone prove a nutritional deficiency, but may be caused by any great number of
conditions or may have functional causes. If these
symptoms persist, they may indicate a condition
other than a vitamin or mineral deficiency.

VITAMIN A

Also known as the anti-infective or anti-ophthalmic
vitamin. Usually measured in U.S.P. units.

NATURAL SOURCES: Colored fruits and vegetables, dairy products, eggs, margarine, fish liver oils, liver.
Builds resistance to infections, especially of the respiratory tract. Helps maintain a healthy condition of the outer layers of many tissues and organs. Promotes growth and vitality. Permits formation of visual purple in the eye, counteracting night blindness and weak eye-sight. Promotes healthy skin. Essential for pregnancy and lactation.

DEFICIENCY: May result in night blindness, increased susceptibility to infections, dry and scaly skin, lack of appetite and vigor, defective teeth and gums, retarded growth.

VITAMIN B1

Thiamin, thiamin chloride. Also known as the anti-neuritic or anti-beriberi vitamin. Measured in milligrams (mg).

NATURAL SOURCES: Dried yeast, rice husks, whole wheat, oatmeal, peanuts, pork, most vegetables, milk.
Promotes growth, aids growth and digestion, essential for normal functioning of nerve tissues, muscles and heart. Repels insects, especially mosquitoes. 100 mg for children; 200–300 for adults.

DEFICIENCY: May lead to loss of appetite, weakness and lassitude, nervous irritability, insomnia, loss of weight, vague aches and pains, mental depression and constipation. In children, deficiency may cause impaired growth.

VITAMIN B2

Riboflavin or vitamin G. Measured in milligrams (mg).

NATURAL SOURCES: Liver, kidney, milk, yeast, cheese, and most B1 sources.
Improves growth, essential for healthy eyes, skin and mouth, promotes general health.

DEFICIENCY: May result in itching and burning of the eyes, cracking of the corners of the lips, inflammation of the mouth, bloodshot eyes, purplish tongue.

VITAMIN B3

Nicotinic acid (niacin), niacinamide (nicotinamide). Measured in milligrams (mg).
The functions and deficiency symptoms of these members of the B complex are similar. Niacinamide is more generally used since it minimizes the burning, flushing and itching of the skin that frequently occurs with nicotinic acid.

NATURAL SOURCES: Liver, lean meat, whole wheat products, yeast, green vegetables, beans.
Important for the proper functioning of the nervous system. Prevents pellagra. Promotes growth. Maintains normal function of the gastrointestinal tract. Necessary for metabolism of sugar. Maintains normal skin conditions. Can reduce blood cholesterol and triglycerides.

DEFICIENCY: May result in pellagra, whose symptoms include inflammation of the skin, tongue; also gastrointestinal disturbance, nervous system dysfunction, headaches, fatigue, mental depression, vague aches and pains, irritability, loss of appetite, neuritis, loss of weight, insomnia, general weakness.

VITAMIN B6

Pyridoxine. Measured in milligrams (mg). If it is designated in micrograms (mcg), remember that it requires 1000 micrograms to equal 1.0 milligram (mg).

NATURAL SOURCES: Meat, fish, wheat germ, egg yolk, cantaloupe, cabbage, milk, yeast.
Aids in food assimilation and in protein and fat metabolism; prevents various nervous and skin disorders, prevents nausea.

DEFICIENCY: May result in nervousness, insomnia, skin eruptions, loss of muscular control. Women who take "the pill" need 4 mg daily.

VITAMIN B12

Commonly known as the "red vitamin" cobalamin. Since it is so effective in small doses, it is the only common vitamin generally expressed in micrograms (mcg).

NATURAL SOURCES: Liver, beef, pork, eggs, milk, cheese.
Helps in the formation and regeneration of red blood cells, thus helping to prevent anemia; promotes growth and increased appetite in children; a general tonic for adults.

DEFICIENCY: May lead to nutritional and pernicious anemias, poor appetite and growth failure in children, tiredness. Women who take "the pill" need 4 mg daily.

VITAMIN B15

Pangamic acid. Controversial member of the B-complex family, highly regarded in Russia.

NATURAL SOURCES: Liver, apricot kernels, rice bran, seeds, brewer's yeast.
Said to improve circulation, energy, aging symptoms and help cure many diseases.

DEFICIENCY: Symptoms are not known.

VITAMIN B17

Laetrile. An especially controversial vitamin since claims have been made for it as a cancer cure.

NATURAL SOURCES: Seeds and kernels.

DEFICIENCY: Not known.

BIOTIN

One of the newly discovered members of the B-complex family. Measured in micrograms (mcg).

NATURAL SOURCES: Yeast. Present in small minute quantities in every living cell.
Growth-promoting factor. Possibly related to metabolism of fats and in the conversion of certain amino-acids.

DEFICIENCY: May lead to extreme exhaustion, drowsiness, muscle pains and loss of appetite; also a type of anemia complicated by a skin disease.

CHOLINE

A member of the vitamin B-complex family. One of the "lipotropic factors." Measured in milligrams (mg).

NATURAL SOURCES: Egg yolks, brain, heart, green leafy vegetables and legumes, yeast, liver and wheat germ. Regulates function of liver; necessary for normal fat metabolism. Minimizes excessive deposits of fat in liver.

DEFICIENCY: May result in cirrhosis and fatty degeneration of liver, hardening of the arteries.

FOLIC ACID

A member of the vitamin B complex. Measured in micrograms (mcg).

NATURAL SOURCES: Deep green leafy vegetables, liver, kidney, yeast.
Essential to the formation of red blood cells by its action on the bone marrow. Aids in protein metabolism and contributes to normal growth.

DEFICIENCY: Nutritional macrocytic anemia. For women who take "the pill," 800 mg are needed daily.

INOSITOL

Another member of the B-complex family. Measured in milligrams (mg).

NATURAL SOURCES: Fruits, nuts, whole grains, milk, meat, yeast.
Similar to that of choline.

DEFICIENCY: Similar to that of choline.

PABA

Para-amino-benzoic acid. Belongs to the B-complex group. Measured in milligrams (mg).

NATURAL SOURCES: Yeast.
A growth-promoting factor, possibly in conjunction with folic acid. In experimental tests on animals, this vitamin when omitted from foods, caused hair to turn white. When restored to the diet, the white hair turned black.

DEFICIENCY: May cause extreme fatigue, eczema, anemia.

CALCIUM PANTOTHENATE

Pantothenic acid. A member of the B-complex family. Measured in milligrams (mg).

NATURAL SOURCES: Liver, kidney, yeast, wheat, bran, peas, crude molasses.
Not clearly defined as yet. Helps in the building of body cells and maintaining normal skin, growth, and development of central nervous system. Required for synthesis of antibodies. Necessary for normal digestive processes. Originally believed to be a factor in restoring gray hair to original color. This function has not been substantiated.

DEFICIENCY: May lead to skin abnormalities, retarded growth, painful and burning feet, dizzy spells, digestive disturbances.

VITAMIN C

Ascorbic acid. Expressed in milligrams (mg), occasionally in units. 1.0 mg equals 20 units.

NATURAL SOURCES: Citrus fruits, berries, greens, cabbages, peppers. (Easily destroyed by cooking.)
Necessary for healthy teeth, gums and bones; strengthens all connective tissue; promotes wound healing; helps promote capillary integrity and prevention of permeability; a very important factor in maintaining sound health and vigor.

DEFICIENCY: May lead to soft gums, tooth decay, loss of appetite, muscular weakness, skin hemorrhages, capillary weakness, anemia.

VITAMIN D

Viosterol, ergosterol, "sunshine vitamin." Measured in U.S.P. units.

NATURAL SOURCES: Fish-liver oils, fat, eggs, milk, butter, sunshine.
Regulates the use of calcium and phosphorus in the body and is therefore necessary for the proper formation of teeth and bones. Very important in infancy and childhood.

DEFICIENCY: May lead to rickets, tooth decay, retarded growth, lack of vigor, muscular weakness.

VITAMIN E

Tocopherol. Available in several different forms. Formerly measured by weight (mg); now generally designated according to its biological activity in International Units (IU).

NATURAL SOURCES: Wheat germ oil, whole wheat, green leaves, vegetable oils, meat, eggs, whole grain cereals, margarine.
Exact function in humans is not yet known. Medical

articles have been published on its value in helping to prevent sterility; in the treatment of threatened abortion; in muscular dystrophy; prevention of calcium deposits in blood vessel walls. Has been used favorably by some doctors in treatment of heart conditions. Much further research needs to be completed before a clear picture of this vitamin will be obtained.

DEFICIENCY: May lead to increased fragility of red blood cells. In experimental animals deficiencies led to loss of reproductive powers and muscular disorders.

VITAMIN F

Unsaturated fatty acids, linoleic acid and linolenic acids.

NATURAL SOURCES: Vegetable oils such as soybean, peanut, safflower, cottonseed, corn and linseed.
A growth-promoting factor; necessary for healthy skin, hair and glands. Promotes the availability of calcium to the cells. Now considered to be important in lowering blood cholesterol and in combating heart disease.

DEFICIENCY: May lead to skin disorders such as eczema.

VITAMIN K

Menadione.

NATURAL SOURCES: Alfalfa and other green plants, soybean oil, egg yolks. Measured in micrograms (mcg), (above 100 mcg RX prescription only in USA).

Essential for the production of prothrombin (a substance which aids the blood in clotting); important to liver function.

DEFICIENCY: Hemorrhages resulting from prolonged blood-clotting time.

VITAMIN P

Citrus bioflavonoids, bioflavonoid complex, hesperidin. Measured in milligrams (mg).

NATURAL SOURCES: Peels and pulp of citrus fruit, especially lemon.
Strengthens walls of capillaries. Prevents vitamin C from being destroyed in the body by oxidation. Beneficial in hypertension, reported to help build resistance in infections and colds.

DEFICIENCY: Capillary fragility. Appearance of purplish spots on skin.

RUTIN

NATURAL SOURCES: Buckwheat. Measured in milligrams (mg).

DEFICIENCY: Similar to that of vitamin P.

THE ESSENTIAL MINERALS AND ALLIED NUTRIENTS

CALCIUM: Builds and maintains bones and teeth; helps blood to clot; aids vitality and endurance; regulates heart rhythm.

COBALT: Stimulant to production of red blood cells; component of vitamin B12; necessary for normal growth and appetite.

COPPER: Necessary for absorption and utilization of iron; formation of red blood cells.

FLUORINE: May decrease incidence of dental caries.

IODINE: Necessary for proper function of thyroid gland; essential for proper growth, energy and metabolism.

IRON: Required in manufacture of hemoglobin; helps carry oxygen in the blood.

MAGNESIUM: Necessary for calcium and vitamin C metabolism; essential for normal functioning of nervous and muscular system.

MANGANESE: Activates various enzymes and other minerals; related to proper utilization of vitamins B1 and E.

MOLYBDENUM: Associated with carbohydrate metabolism.

PHOSPHORUS: Needed for normal bone and tooth structure. Interrelated with action of calcium and vitamin D.

POTASSIUM: Necessary for normal muscle tone, nerves, heart action and enzyme reactions.

SULFUR: Vital to good skin, hair and nails.

ZINC: Helps normal tissue function, protein and carbohydrate metabolism.

Some important vitamins and what they do ———————————

Vitamin A

It is a fat soluble vitamin measured in USP (United States Pharmacopoeia) units, IU (International Units) and RE (Retinol Equivalents).

It occurs in two forms—preformed vitamin A, called retinol (found only in foods of animal origin), and provitamin A, known as carotene (provided by foods of both plant and animal origin).

10,000 IU daily is the average adult dosage, though the need increases with greater body weight.

Vitamin A is essential to counteract night blindness, weak eyesight and aid in the treatment of many eye disorders. It builds resistance to respiratory infections and shortens the duration of diseases.

This vitamin keeps the outer layers of your tissues and organs healthy.

More than 100,000 IU daily, if taken for many months can produce toxic effects in adults. More than 18,500 IU daily can produce the same effect in infants.

The B-complex group

The B-complex group of vitamins consists of:
Vitamin B1 (or thiamin)
Vitamin B2 (or riboflavin)
Vitamin B3 (or niacin, niacinamide)
Vitamin B6 (or pyridoxine)
Vitamin B12 (or cyanocobalamin, cobalamin)
Folic acid (or folacin, pteroylglutamic acid)
D-calcium pantothenate
Pantothenic acid (pantothenate, panthenol)
Biotin (or D-biotin)
Para-amino-benzoic acid (or PABA)
Choline
Inositol
Vitamin B15 (or calcium pangamate or pangamic acid)
Vitamin B17 (or amygdalin or laetrile)

The B-complex vitamins help release energy from food, thus increasing the available body energy to help fight fatigue. Research indicates that deficiency of B vitamins may lead to irritability, nervousness, fear and even depression. Therefore, this is a group of vitamins necessary for calm nerves and mental stability. During stress conditions (disease, anxiety, trauma, post surgery) many doctors prescribe a "Stress Formula" which incorporates the B complex with vitamin C.

B-complex vitamins help form healthy red blood cells that supply oxygen to the tissue. They can be used to relieve insomnia, neuritis, anemia and high cholesterol.

Leading members of the vitamin B complex

Choline

In 1846, N. T. Gobley discovered a substance from egg yolk which contained glycerol, fatty acids (linoleic and linolenic acids), phosphorus and nitrogen. He called it lecithin.

In 1932, Dr. C. H. Best (co-discoverer of insulin) at the University of Toronto made the discovery that choline was important to nutrition. Further research proved that choline has a definite relationship to the metabolism of fats.

In 1968, Strecker isolated a nitrogenous base from lecithin which he called choline.

Choline is required by the thymus gland; it is needed for lactation and especially important for kidney and liver function. In some cases, choline has brought about vast improvement in cases of cirrhosis of the liver caused by alcoholism. Today, choline is being prescribed for such diverse ailments as: gallbladder trouble, diabetes, muscular dystrophy, glaucoma and arteriosclerosis. The best source of choline is still lecithin.

Inositol

In 1940, D. W. Wooley isolated inositol from liver. In subsequent experiments, it was found to recover hair in mice after they had lost it on certain other diets. Other reports showed inositol was a growth stimulative to rats, chicks and dogs. Later an important relationship was established linking inositol, human metabolism and cholesterol.

Inositol has proved valuable to man as an auxiliary to vitamin E, helping to facilitate its actions in the treatment of muscular dystrophy. Inositol is also used in therapy of other nerve and muscle disorders, such as multiple sclerosis and cerebral palsy. However, there is still much to be learned about inositol.

Adelle Davis, in her book *Let's Get Well*, states that increasing the intake of protein, particularly of liver, wheat germ, and yeast, and supplementing the diet with a teaspoon of inositol (1000 mg) daily usually stops hair loss.

Both choline and inositol are lipotropics [fat loving], formidable opponents of cholesterol and viruses. (*See* p. 85)

Vitamin B6

Vitamin B6, or pyridoxine, is becoming more and more important because a growing number of scientific-clinical documentation is showing its use in the circulatory system and in the functioning of the nervous and musculo-skeletal systems.

Without vitamin B6, protein cannot be utilized properly by the body; therefore, a high protein diet should include additional B6. It also helps utilize fats and carbohydrates and is essential to maintain and repair body tissues.

In Dr. John M. Ellis's and James Presley's book, *Vitamin B6, The Doctor's Report*, published by Harper & Row, Inc., eight disease conditions in which B6 therapy has been used successfully were discussed. These include tingling fingers, muscle spasms during the night, leg cramps, numbness in the hands and severe pain of the arms, shoulders and chest.

Dr. Ellis states that it was discovered in hospitals and clinics that B6 relieves certain forms of neuritis in the feet, arms, legs and hands. He also showed that edema (an excessive accumulation of fluid in the tissues) can be drastically reduced by vitamin B6.

"The Amazing Cider Vinegar, Lecithin, Kelp plus B6 Diet" from *The Natural Way to Super Beauty* by Mary Ann Crenshaw (Dell, 1981) utilizes vitamin B6 for its anti-edema properties.

Dr. Ellis learned that hormones require an increased amount of B6 or become toxic in the absence of it. This is significant for pregnant and menopausal women, as well as for millions of women taking birth control pills. They should take at least 25–30 mg of B6, 4 mg of B12 and 800 mg of folic acid daily. Also, vitamin C is depleted by a minimum of 100 mg daily. Low vitamin C levels may account for increased susceptibility to blood-clotting.

B15 pangamate
(Calcium pangamate, pangamic acid)

What does it do?
1. It increases the supply of oxygen in the blood.
2. According to the Russians it:
   A. Extends cell life spans.
   B. Stimulates immune response.
   C. Is involved in energy transport.
   D. Detoxifies pollutants.
   E. Is involved in protein synthesis.
   F. Speeds recovery from fatigue.
   G. Regulates the blood levels of steroids.

The conditions that can be treated by B15 (according to the Russians)

Aging	Hepatitis
Alcoholism	High blood pressure
Allergies	Jaundice
Autism	Mild poisoning
Cirrhosis	Minimal brain dysfunction
Dermatitis	Neuralgia
Diabetes	Neuritis
Drug addiction	Schizophrenia
Gangrene	Sciatica
Glaucoma	Senility
Heart disease	

B15 and alcoholism

According to Dr. I. V. Strelchuk of the Central Research Institute of Forensic Psychiatry in Moscow, B15 neutralizes the craving for alcohol by the alcoholic. After one month of pangamate treatment, Russian alcoholics cannot stand the sight of vodka. B15 also protects against cirrhosis of the liver. Dr. Robert Atkins *(Super Energy Diet)* has stated that B15 lessens the severity of a hangover from alcohol.

WHO TAKES IT?

Soviet athletes eat B15 like candy. Dick Gregory, Gary Null, Muhammad Ali, all take the supplement.

DOSAGE

B15 usually comes in 50 mg tablet strength. The average dose is one to three tablets daily, with or after meals.

Your author takes one 50 mg tablet in the morning with breakfast and one tablet in the evening with dinner.

Vitamin C

Vitamin C is one of the most important vitamins our bodies require. Since man has lost the ability to manufacture his own vitamin C, he must replace this precious vitamin every day of his life or suffer the consequences.

Vitamin C is essential for the formation of collagen in the body; collagen is a protein substance which cements together the cells needed to make tissue.

Collagen is important to the body because:

1. It is necessary for structural soundness of bones, teeth, connective tissue, cartilage and capillary walls.
2. It plays a role in wound and burn healing. It is necessary for the formation of healthy connective tissue used by the body to knit together a wound or burn.
3. It may play an important role in protecting the body from infection. A current theory holds that healthy collagen means stronger tissue which enables the body to resist invasion by disease micro-organisms.

The body's need for vitamin C appears to increase greatly during stress conditions. Emotional stress, extremely low environmental temperature, fever and infections are all stress conditions. Women taking birth control pills need an extra 100 mg of C a day.

The vitamin C content of white blood cells destroys invading micro-organisms. Vitamin C has antihistamine action, which may explain some recent findings regarding the pharmacological effect or reducing morbidity from acute respiratory illness.

According to Dr. Arend Bouhays, Yale University Lung Research Center, New Haven, Connecticut: "Oral administration of 500 mg of vitamin C reduces the airway constriction induced by inhalation of histamine in healthy adults." Vitamin C also affords protection against the airway-constrictor effects of certain textile dusts that act through release of histamine in the lungs, Dr. Bouhays added. If histamine plays a part in promoting mucosal inflammation in acute respiratory illness, Dr. Bouhays speculates, then the antihistamine action of vitamin C might explain in part the reduced symptoms and duration of the illnesses.

What is the best way to take vitamin C?

People are becoming more aware of the need to supplement their diets with extra vitamin C. Unfortunately, most people think that by taking an ordinary vitamin C tablet in the morning with their breakfast, they will be covered for the rest of the day. Actually, the vitamin C is metabolized and any excess is excreted in about two hours, depending on the quantity of food in the stomach.

It is very important to maintain a constant high level of vitamin C in the blood stream at all times, since it can be destroyed by stress and/or carbon monoxide from exhaust fumes. The problem we face is how?

Fortunately, modern science has solved this problem by the invention of time release vitamin C tablets. These tablets slowly release C into our blood stream for eight to twelve hours, depending on individual body chemistry. Thus by taking a tablet at breakfast, at midafternoon and at bedtime, we can be assured that we are constantly protected.

How long will vitamin C last on my shelf?

Long-term and short-term tests indicate that, under normal storage conditions, commercial vitamin C tablets are stable for periods in excess of five years (95 percent potency retention).

Minute amounts of breakdown products formed under various storage conditions reportedly do not present any dietary hazard.

This was reported by Dr. S. H. Rubin, E. De-Ritter, and J. B. Johnson, of Hoffman-La Roche, at a meeting of the APHA Academy of Pharmaceutical Sciences in Atlanta, Georgia, on November 18, 1975.

Do smokers need more vitamin C?

Over a two-year period, researchers studied smokers and nonsmokers of ages 20 to 64. They gathered data on 812 male nonsmokers, 1,243 male smokers, 1,526 female nonsmokers, and 1,091 female smokers.

The results clearly showed that cigarette smokers with dietary vitamin C intakes comparable to those of nonsmokers have lower blood serum vitamin C than nonsmokers. In another study, heavy cigarette smokers had as much as 40 percent lower blood plasma levels than nonsmokers. One cigarette destroys at least 25 mg of vitamin C.

Dr. Omer Pelletier, research scientist in the Bureau of Nutritional Sciences, Food Directorate, Health Protection Branch in Ottawa, Canada reported these findings to the second conference on vitamin C sponsored by the New York Academy of Sciences.

Research shows the benefits of vitamin C

1. *Against allergies*: Dr. James A. Jackson states, "vitamin C can be very effective in the treatment of many allergies. It may be used alone or with other agents." Large doses of vitamin C can decrease allergic symptoms, especially runny nose and cough.

    (*Ascorbic Acid versus Allergies*, Dr. James A. Jackson, 1972.)

    Mechanism of action: vitamin C inhibits the airway constriction effect of histamine in healthy human subjects (works as an antihistamine). The dosage varies from 500 mg up to 5000 mg in divided doses.

2. *Against asthma*: Dr. E. Zuskin noted in the *Journal of Allergy and Clinical Immunology* that vitamin C could diminish, if not prevent completely, the symptoms of byssinosis, a lung disease which strikes textile workers who breathe fiber dust.

    (Zuskin, E., et al., "Inhibition of Histamine-Induced Airway Constriction by Ascorbic Acid," *Journal of Allergy and Clinical Immunology*, P: 218–226, 1973.)

    The mechanism of action is that vitamin C inhibits the airway constriction effect of histamine (works as an antihistamine). The dosage used was 250 mg every three hours throughout the day.

3. *Against arteriosclerosis* (Hardening of the arteries): Vitamin C helps reduce cholesterol levels and possibly slows arteriosclerosis. Sixty geriatric patients took 1–3 grams of vitamin C for

thirty months. During that time none had a heart attack, although each had a history of heart trouble. Of the 60, 83 percent experienced a mild to impressive improvement in their symptoms. The dosage was 1–3 grams daily in divided doses.

(Spittle, C. R., "Arteriosclerosis and Vitamin C," *Lancet* 2: 1280–1283, 1971.)

4. *Against colds*

A. Dr. T. W. Anderson, writing in the *Canadian Medical Association Journal,* discovered that patients taking 1000 mg of vitamin C or 1 gram every day (and increasing that dose to 4 grams at the onset of a cold) had a 9 percent reduction in colds frequency and 14 percent reduction in sick days.

(Anderson, T. W., et al., "Vitamin C and the Common Cold: A Double Blind Trial," *CMA Journal* 107: 503–508, 1972.)

B. Dr. John Colehan, in the *New England Journal of Medicine* in 1974 discovered that although they could not prevent the incidence of colds in a Navajo Indian boarding school, they could significantly decrease the sick days due to respiratory illness by 28–34 percent at a dose of 1000 to 2000 mg of vitamin C every day. They also found that vitamin C decreased by 30 percent the incidence of non-cold-related illness.

(Colehan, John L., et al., "Vitamin C Prophylaxis in a Boarding School," *New England Journal of Medicine*, 290: 6–10, 1974.)

C. In 1973 a study was carried out in a Dublin, Ireland, boarding school which showed sex differences in response to vitamin C treatment. Girls received the rather small dose of 500 mg vitamin C and showed that the severity and intensity of their cold symptoms were reduced by 50 percent. Boys showed lower percentages.

(Wilson, C. W. M. and Loh, H. S., "Common Cold and Vitamin C," *Lancet*, P. 638, 1973.)

D. Dr. Linus Pauling in his book *Vitamin C and the Common Cold* suggests the dosage of vitamin C for everyone is between 1 gram and 2 grams (2000 mg) daily. When a cold starts, he suggests 5 to 10 grams.

(*Vitamin C and the Common Cold*, Dr. Linus Pauling, W. H. Freeman, 1971.)

5. *Against gallstones*: Guinea pigs fed a diet deficient in vitamin C tend to accumulate cholesterol in their livers. This situation may stimulate the formation of gallstones.

(Ginter, E., "Vitamin C Deficiency and Gallstone Formation," *Lancet*, 2: 1198–1199, 1971.)

6. *Lemon bioflavonoids* or vitamin P can help vitamin C to work even better. A deficiency of bioflavonoids can lead to bleeding gums, a very common disorder among Americans. Many dentists recommend this food supplement.

Capillary fragility, or bruising, another very common occurrence among women, can be cleared up with a combination of vitamin C and lemon bioflavonoids.

Rutin, derived from buckwheat and hesperidin, is part of the C complex and works with vitamin C to make it more beneficial.

Vitamin D (calciferol, viosterol, ergosterol, the "sunshine vitamin")

It is a fat soluble vitamin, acquired through sunlight

or diet. (Ultraviolet sun rays act on the oils of the skin to produce the vitamin, which is then absorbed into the body.) Measured in International Units (IU).

The RDA for adults is 400 IU daily.

Vitamin D is necessary for the body to properly utilize calcium and phosphorus which are both important for strong bones and teeth. Taken with vitamin A and C it can aid in preventing colds.

Five thousand to 150,000 IU daily over an extended period can produce toxic effects in adults. Thirty thousand IU to babies and more than 45,000 IU to children can easily produce symptoms of toxicity.

Vitamin E

In 1922, at the University of California, a substance was found to be an anti-sterility factor. Two years later, this substance was named vitamin E. Vitamin E was assigned its chemical name, tocopherol, around 1936, when it was isolated from wheat germ oil. Tocopherol comes from the Greek "taco," meaning childbirth, and "phero," meaning to bring forth. All research up to the present indicates that only *alpha* tocopherol is biologically active. Since alpha tocopherol is unstable, it has been stabilized with acetic acid to produce alpha tocopherol acetate, which converts in the body to alpha tocopherol.

Dr. A. L. Tappel, of the University of California at Davis published his work on the antioxidant properties of vitamin E in the aging process in 1963. Most of the vitamin E research being conducted is

31

devoted to its antioxidant properties. Recent studies indicate vitamin E plays a role in the protection of vitamin A. A process of oxygen combining with other substances (oxidation) is a normal and natural process wherever oxygen is available from other nutrients or from transformations that take place in metabolism. The presence of vitamin E reduces the body's requirement for oxygen.

Oxidation during metabolism is necessary for the proper utilization of various nutrients. When the body has too much of a certain substance, it may not be able to excrete all of the oxidized end products fast enough and the spoiled matter remains in the system longer. The longer these undesirable substances remain in the system, the greater the chances that they will combine with other substances and cause trouble. Rapid destruction of polyunsaturated fatty acids as well as other fats is called lipid peroxidation. Lipid peroxidation causes free radicals to form and the combination of peroxidation and free cellular radicals damages the cell—thus the aging process. Vitamin E as an antioxidant can slow down the oxidation of fats and oils, and enhance the activity of vitamin A.

Vitamins A and E can protect lungs against air pollution. Vitamin E is a natural anticoagulant, dissolving blood clots safely. Vitamin E can also permeate the tiny capillaries and assist in bringing nourishment to all body cells and thereby supply oxygen to the muscles (especially the heart muscles). A vitamin E deficiency decreases the production of all pituitary hormones; of ACTH, essential to stimulate the adrenals, and the hormones which stimulate the thyroid and sex glands.

Vitamin E has also been used successfully in treating burns. It accelerates the healing rate of burns and lessens the formation of scar tissue. When applied to the skin, the antioxidizing effect of vitamin E prevents bacteria from growing and reduces thereby the chances of unwanted odors.

Vitamin E seems to prevent undesirable excessive scarring of the heart after an infarct, while it promotes a strong "patch" scar during the healing process.

Vitamin E is a vasodilator. It allows a greater flexibility in cells and muscles, preventing hardening of the arteries. Athletes have found greater stamina resulting from the vasodilating quality of vitamin E. These are the advantages:

Vitamin E seems to be an anti-clotting agent that helps prevent blood clots in arteries and veins, helps dissolve existing clots (fibrinolytic activity), increases the blood's available oxygen (i.e., improves the transportation of oxygen by the red blood cells), reduces the need of the heart for oxygen by making the heart become a more efficient pump, and seems to be a vasodilator (capillary) developing collateral blood vessels to facilitate circulation. It also improves capillary permeability (ability to pass through).

Diabetics have been found to be able to reduce their insulin levels when given vitamin E. If you are diabetic, check with your doctor.

Dr. Wilfrid Shute, a pioneer in the use of vitamin E, and author of *The Complete Vitamin E Book* (Keats, 1975), recommended 800 IU of E for the average male and 400 for the average female until recently; he now says that environmental threats have made it desirable for people not subject to high blood pressure or with rheumatic fever in their histories to take 1600 IUs a day.

Minerals and Elements——
*The Cinderella supplements*_____

I like to call minerals the Cinderella supplements
of the world of nutrition. Very few people realize
that vitamins cannot function without the aid of
minerals.

Minerals are synergistic, i.e., they work better
together than individually. They work in partner-
ship with hormones, enzymes and vitamins. They
are required to build and maintain the structure of
the body.

Minerals are necessary for carbohydrates, proteins and fats to be broken down in digestion and
built into cells and transformed into energy. Those
that are currently considered essential for human
nutrition are: calcium, phosphorus, iron, potassium,
sodium, iodine and magnesium. Processed or refined foods (for example: white flour and white
sugar) are almost devoid of all trace minerals.

CALCIUM

Calcium is by far the most important mineral the body requires, yet calcium deficiency is more prevalent than that of any other mineral. The adult body contains three to four pounds of calcium, 99 percent of which is in bones and teeth. (From the age of 9, the diets of girls and women may lack as much as 25–30 percent of the calcium they need.) Symptoms of calcium deficiencies are stunted growth, decayed teeth, and nervousness. Without sufficient calcium in the bloodstream, nerves cannot send messages and therefore cause tension. Fingertapping, impatience and quick temper can be signs of calcium deficiencies. Calcium can only be assimilated by getting plenty of phosphorus, iodine, vitamin A, vitamin B, vitamin F and vitamin D. Adequate hydrochloric acid in the stomach is also necessary for the absorption of calcium.

Since it is so concentrated in the bones and teeth, only 1 percent circulates in body fluids and tissues. Calcium is needed for normal blood coagulation or clotting, to activate enzymes (digestive juices) and to regulate fluid passages throughout cellular walls. It is required for every heartbeat. An inadequate calcium intake means that some calcium is stored in the ends of the bones. Under stress situations this reserve storage is used. If the body has no reserve calcium, then it is seized from the bone structure, usually the spinal and pelvic bones.

Calcium and phosphorus must exist in a two-to-one ratio in the body, that is, two parts calcium and one part phosphorus. Vitamin D helps to normalize and maintain a good balance of calcium and phosphorus. Also, the two-to-one relationship is necessary for magnesium and calcium—two parts calcium to one part magnesium.

Calcium is vital to the nerves of the body. Calcium also maintains the delicate acid-alkaline body balance. The best calcium source is bone meal. The calcium-phosphorus balance is built in.

CHLORINE

This element works with sodium and potassium to set up conditions for the irritability and contractility of the muscle tissue and the sending of messages through the nervous system.

COPPER

Copper works as a catalyst in the formation of red blood cells. Copper is also present in the hemoglobin molecule. Copper is essential before iron can be utilized. Copper is needed to prevent anemia.

FLUORINE

An element that helps protect teeth from decay.

IODINE

The most important fact about iodine is that a deficiency of it can cause goiter—a swelling of the thyroid gland. Kelp is a good source of natural iodine. Seafoods are very high in iodine.

IRON

Women need more iron than men because of the loss of blood during the menstrual cycle. Pregnancy and breastfeeding also increase the body's demand for iron. The pregnant woman transfers iron to the growing fetus and to the placenta. This transfer of iron is heaviest during the last three months of pregnancy.

Iron is the second most deficient mineral in the human body. Iron is the prime factor in anemia prevention, the key factor in healthy blood. It is the essential ingredient in hemoglobin—the red coloring matter in blood. Without iron, the blood could not carry oxygen to the tissues. Without oxygen, the body tissues die.

Dangers of vegetarianism

Many people run the risk of an iron-poor diet when they restrict their food intake in an effort to lose weight. Vegetarian diets also increase the likelihood that the body's need for iron will not be met. If you believe in vegetarianism, double check your diet. Consider the advantages of iron supplements as health insurance.

The symptoms of anemia

The most noticeable warning sign of anemia is fatigue. If you are getting plenty of rest, but still feel tired and lacking in energy, your body could be telling you that you are becoming anemic.

The hair, skin and nails also show the effects of anemia. The skin tends to wrinkle more. Fingernails and toenails become brittle and break easily, and become tender. Hair becomes dry and lacks luster. Skin color becomes paler, even pasty and gray. The mouth and tongue begin to feel sore and tender.

Fortunately, the treatment of iron-deficiency

anemia is as simple as checking with your doctor and taking iron supplements by mouth.

Copper, cobalt, manganese and vitamin C are necessary to assimilate iron. B-complex vitamins, such as B1, B6, biotin, folic acid and B12, all work with iron to produce rich red blood. Inorganic iron—ferrous sulfate—destroys vitamin E, and if you are taking both, space them 8 hours apart. Organic iron—ferrous gluconate, ferrous citrate or ferrous peptonate—has no effect on vitamin E.

MAGNESIUM

Dr. Hans Selye of McGill University calls this mineral the anti-stress mineral. He has saved animals under great stress by giving them protective amounts of magnesium. Those animals without the protective mineral died of heart damage. Calcium and magnesium are found in perfect balance in nature for optimum absorption in dolomite. In controlled studies of rats, it was found that magnesium was necessary to prevent calcium deposits, kidney stones and gallstones.

MANGANESE

This mineral functions in blood formation and is an activator of the urea.

POTASSIUM

Potassium is an essential mineral, like calcium and phosphorus. It is needed in somewhat the same quantities as magnesium. There must be a proper balance between sodium, calcium and potassium.

Potassium is needed in many functions, but especially for heart rhythm. Aided by sodium, it also assists the cells in the selection of food particles. Both potassium and sodium help to pull the particles out of the blood and both minerals aid the cells in the elimination of wastes. Potassium attracts the nourishment that the cells need from the bloodstream.

Organic potassium—the gluconate, the citrate, the fumerate—is preferable to the inorganic—the sulfate (alum), the chloride, the oxide and carbonate, etc. Natural sources for potassium are primarily green leafy vegetables. Most people do not eat enough of these. Unfortunately, they are not an adequate source for any potent supply; supplements are needed.

Ninety-eight percent of the total body potassium is found inside the cells, while the remaining 2 percent is distributed between the bloodstream and other body fluids. Potassium depletion is common in long fasts, chronic disease characterized by weight loss, and muscle atrophy. Major surgery or other major trauma such as burns, fractures, severe muscle damage or severe diarrhea also cause potassium loss.

But the most common cause today is man-made. It is the use of diuretic drugs ("water pills"). They are used in the treatment of edema and hypertension (high blood pressure). The problem is so common that many physicians routinely prescribe potassium supplements for long periods of time. A special supplement is needed—if you take a diuretic, consult your doctor. Other causes of potassium loss are the use of the steroid drugs, cortisone and ACTH and chronic stress, which causes constant release of certain hormones.

The symptoms of potassium loss are: fatigue, muscle weakness, paralysis and frequent urination.

SODIUM

Sodium helps to balance the acid-base relationship in the body. It is needed to keep calcium in solution.

SELENIUM

Selenium's reputation is growing fast; it seems to solve such problems as:

Can it help dandruff?
Is there a relationship between selenium content in human blood and the cancer death rate?
How does it work with vitamin E?
Can it help prostate problems?

In 1957, Dr. Klaus Schwarz and Dr. C. M. Katz established that selenium is essential to life, even though it is needed in very small quantities. A good recommended dosage of selenium is between 50 mcg to 100 mcg daily, not to exceed 200 mcg daily.

By processing grain, the miller robs 75 percent of its selenium content to produce white flour. Today, there is a new yeast which contains 100 or more times the ordinary level of selenium than is usually present in yeast.

Your doctor would probably recommend a dandruff shampoo that contains selenium if you asked him. These commercial shampoos, either the blue or the yellow, may help dandruff by correcting the system's deficiency of selenium. It could be possible to overcome dandruff by taking selenium supplements!

Vitamin E and selenium are synergistic. The two

Selenium Concentration in Human Blood & Human Cancer Death Rate in Various Cities 1962—66

City	Blood Selenium concentration mcg/100 ml	Cancer deaths per 100,000
Rapid City, S.D.	25.6	94.0
Cheyenne, Wyo.	23.4	104.0
Spokane, Wash.	23.0	179.0
Fargo, N.D.	21.7	142.0
Little Rock, Ark.	20.1	176.0
Phoenix, Ariz.	19.7	126.7
Meridian, Miss.	19.5	125.0
Missoula, Mont.	19.4	174.0
El Paso, Tex.	19.2	119.0
Jacksonville, Fla.	18.8	199.0
Red Bluff, Calif. (Tehama Co.)	18.2	176.0
Geneva, N.Y.	18.2	172.0
Billings, Mont.	18.0	138.0
Montpelier, Vt. (Wash. Co.)	18.0	164.0
Lubbock, Tex.	17.8	115.0
Lafayette, La.	17.6	145.0
Canandaigua, N.Y.	15.7	188.0
(Ontario Co.)	17.6	168.0
Muncie, Ind.	15.8	169.0
Lima, Ohio	15.7	188.0

Shamberger and Willis, *CRC Reviews*, June 1971.

It is interesting to observe that in Rapid City, S.D., which has the highest blood levels of selenium in any municipality in the U.S., the cancer death rate is the lowest in the country. Coincidence? Maybe!

together are stronger than the sum of their equal parts.

Dr. Richard Passwater says that researchers have already confirmed that if mice are fed antioxidant nutrients, such as vitamin E and C and selenium, and then given a typical carcinogen which tends to induce stomach cancer or skin cancer in mice within four months, 90 percent of these animals will not come down with cancer (*Cancer and Its Nutritional Therapies*, Keats, 1978). In other words, selenium seems to help neutralize some carcinogens.

Males should be especially interested in selenium, as they may have a greater need for it than females. Almost half of a male's total selenium supply concentrates in the testicles and portions of the seminal ducts adjacent to the prostate glands. Selenium is lost in the semen.

It seems to this writer that, with all the current research findings on selenium, we have only just begun to learn about this "miracle element."

SULFUR

Sulfur is a blood conditioner and cleanser. It aids the liver in absorbing the other minerals. Referred to as the beauty mineral, it has been known to make the difference between stringy or shimmery hair, brittle or beautiful nails, and, coupled with vitamins A and D, to play a major part in skin texture integrity.

ZINC

Think of zinc as a traffic policeman, directing and overseeing the efficient flow of body processes, the maintenance of enzyme systems and the integrity of our cells. It is a tiny but powerful catalyst which is absolutely essential for most integral body functions.

Zinc is a trace mineral found in such small amounts in our bodies that it has been called a micronutrient. It is found in the thyroid gland, hair, finger and toenails, nervous system, liver, bones, pancreas, kidney, pituitary glands, blood and in the male reproductive fluid or semen. It is the prime element in male hormone production. Zinc is a constituent of insulin, which is necessary for the utilization of sugar. It also assists food absorption through the intestinal wall.

Most zinc available in foods is lost in processing. For example, 80 percent of the zinc in white bread is destroyed by processing.

Zinc governs the contractility of our muscles, stabilizes blood and maintains the relationship of acidity and alkalinity in the blood and other fluids. Its use exerts a normalizing effect upon the prostate and a lack of the mineral can produce testicular atrophy and prostate trouble.

Zinc is essential for the synthesis of protein and in the action of many enzymes. A lack of zinc can cause increased fatigue, susceptibility to infection and injury and a slowdown in alertness and scholastic achievement.

Henry A. Schroeder, M.D. of Dartmouth Medical School, the world's leading authority on trace minerals, believed that elderly people should take at least 10 mg of zinc daily. He further thinks that pregnant women, or those who take the birth control pill, need supplemental zinc, since both conditions can result in deficiency.

(Trace Elements and Man, Devin-Adair, 1973).

Dr. Carl C. Pfeiffer in *Mental and Elemental Nutrients* (Keats, 1977), relates zinc deficiency to mental illnesses such as schizophrenia, (which he treats with zinc and vitamin B6), senile dementia and other psychoses. White spots or bands on fingernails, he says, may indicate zinc deficiency.

Foods rich in zinc include brewer's yeast, bone meal, beans, pumpkin and sunflower seeds, wheat germ, fertile eggs, fish and meat. Liver is an exceptional source.

How to improve your nutrition

The success of any program of nutritional therapy is founded upon a sound daily diet. In the case of disease or deficiency conditions, this is especially important since the body must receive substantial quantities of high quality "building blocks" such as protein to facilitate the vitamins and minerals in their action. Eliminate food items which contribute little or nothing to nutritional or physical status. Emphasize those which are beneficial.

What to eliminate

Sugar: White and brown and products containing any refined sugar. Sugar substitutes (saccharin, cyclamate). Honey or molasses may be used sparingly.

Refined Flours: White, partially refined, bleached and any products such as pastry, cookies, cakes or breads containing flours of this type.

Refined Grains: Hot and cold breakfast cereals and cereal products unless prepared from unprocessed whole grain. Moderate use of Granola or Roman Meal type products is acceptable. White rice and blanched or de-germed grains.

Pasta: Macaroni, noodles, spaghetti and related items.

Vegetables: Whole potatoes, corn, beans other than green or wax, and peas do not have to be eliminated but should be used sparingly.

Dessert: Virtually all except prepared dietetic varieties or homemade types without added sugar such as fresh fruit cups.

Beverages: Alcoholic beverages, soft drinks, strong tea and coffee.

Miscellaneous: All snack foods, chips, candy products, ice cream and related items. French fries and deep fried foods, especially when prepared in batter.

Dried Fruits: All dried fruits including apricots, raisins, dates, etc.

Other Fruits: Bananas, grapes, cherries, mangoes, avocados. All canned fruits with syrup added unless this is rinsed off with water.

*These categories should only be eliminated by persons following therapeutic dietary programs. [Example: low cholesterol, diabetic, hypoglycemic, low calorie, etc.]

What to increase or feature

Dairy Products: Milk (2 percent, skimmed, raw, powder), buttermilk, yogurt (unflavored), cottage cheese, cheddar and other non-processed cheeses.

Grain Products: Wheat germ, bran, wholegrain cereals and bread, full fat soy flour, and other items prepared from whole oats, rye, barley, etc. Brown or converted rice.

Meat: All forms may be liberally consumed provided all visible fat is removed prior to cooking. Organ meats, fowl, and eggs are excellent. Ham, sausages, weiners, and most canned meat should be avoided if possible.

Seafood: All types of fish excluding salmon, herring, and fish canned in oil. Clams, oysters and other shellfish are excellent.

Nuts and Seeds: Nuts and seeds of all varieties may be consumed daily in moderate amounts provided they are unroasted, unsalted, and without added oil. Especially good are toasted soybeans, raw almonds, cashews, pumpkin and sunflower seeds.

Vegetables: All vegetables except those listed under "Eliminate" should be used regularly and in abundance. Maximum benefit is obtained from fresh or frozen rather than canned varieties. Emphasis should be placed on leafy green vegetables and the regular use of salads.

Fruit: All types except those listed under "Eliminate." Use regularly.

Beverages: All fruit and vegetable juices except grape, prune and those with added sugar. Weak tea, herbal teas, decaffeinated coffee, and the beverages listed under "Dairy Products" are acceptable.

Refined White Table Sugar Content of America's Leading Cereals by Weight

Cereal	% of sugar	Cereal	% of sugar
All Bran	19	Honey Comb	37
Alpha Bits	38	KIX	5
Apple Jacks	55	Life	16
Cap'n Crunch	40	Lucky Charms	42
Cheerios	3	Oatmeal	0
Chex	4	100% Bran	21
Cocoa Pebbles	43	Product 19	10
Cocoa Puffs	33	Quaker 100%	
Concentrate	9	Natural Cereal	21
Cookie Crisp	44	Raisin Bran	30
Corn Flakes	5	Rice Krispies	8
Count Chocula	40	Shredded Wheat	1
Crazy Cow	40	Special K	5
C.W. Post	29	Sugar Frosted Flakes	41
Farina	0	Sugar Smacks	56
40% Bran	13	Super Sugar Crisp	46
Franken Berry	44	Total	8
Fruit Loops	48	Trix	36
Frosted Mini-Wheats	26	Wheatena	0
Fruity Pebbles	43	Wheat Germ	0
Golden Grahams	30	Wheaties	8
Grape-Nuts	7		

*Source *Earl Mindell's Vitamin Bible for Your Kids*. New York: Rawson-Wade, 1981.

Do you eat too much sugar?

Here are the approximate amounts of refined sugar (added sugar, in addition to the sugar naturally present) hidden in popular foods.

Food Item	Size Portion	Approximate Sugar Content in Teaspoonful of Granulated Sugar
Beverages		
cola drinks	1 (6 oz bottle or glass)	3½
cordials	1 (¾ oz glass)	1½
ginger ale	6 oz	5
highball	1 (6 oz glass)	2½
Orangeade	1 (8 oz glass)	5
root beer	1 (10 oz bottle)	4½
Seven-Up	1 (6 oz bottle or glass)	3¾
soda pop	1 (8 oz bottle)	5
sweet cider	1 cup	6
whiskey sour	1 (3 oz glass)	1½
Cakes and Cookies		
angel food	1 (4 oz piece)	7
apple sauce cake	1 (4 oz piece)	5½
banana cake	1 (2 oz piece)	2
cheese cake	1 (4 oz piece)	2
choc. cake (plain)	1 (4 oz piece)	6
choc. cake (iced)	1 (4 oz piece)	10
coffee cake	1 (4 oz piece)	4½
cup cake (iced)	1	6
fruit cake	1 (4 oz piece)	5
jelly roll	1 (2 oz piece)	2½
orange cake	1 (4 oz piece)	4
pound cake	1 (4 oz piece)	5
sponge cake	1 (1 oz piece)	2
brownies (unfrosted)	1 (¾ oz)	3
chocolate cookies	1	1½
Fig Newtons	1	5
gingersnaps	1	3
macaroons	1	6

Food Item	Size Portion	Approximate Sugar Content in Teaspoonful of Granulated Sugar
nut cookies	1	1½
oatmeal cookies	1	2
sugar cookies	1	1½
chocolate eclair	1	7
cream puff	1	2
doughnut (plain)	1	3
doughnut (glazed)	1	6

Candies

average choc. milk bar	1 (1½ oz)	2½
chewing gum	1 stick	½
chocolate cream	1 piece	2
butterscotch chew	1 piece	1
chocolate mints	1 piece	2
fudge	1 oz square	4½
gumdrop	1	2
hard candy	4 oz	20
Lifesavers	1	⅓
peanut brittle	1 oz	3½

Canned Fruits and Juices

canned apricots	4 halves and 1 T syrup	3½
canned fruit juices (sweet)	½ cup	2
canned peaches	2 halves and 1 T syrup	3½
fruit salad	½ cup	3½
fruit syrup	2 T	2½
stewed fruits	½ cup	2

Dairy Products

ice cream	⅓ pt (3½ oz)	3½
ice cream cone	1	3½
ice cream soda	1	5
ice cream sundae	1	7
malted milk shake	1 (10 oz glass)	5

Food Item	Size Portion	Approximate Sugar Content in Teaspoonful of Granulated Sugar
Jams and Jellies		
apple butter	1 T	1
jelly	1 T	4–6
orange marmalade	1 T	4–6
peach butter	1 T	1
strawberry jam	1 T	4
Desserts, Miscellaneous		
apple cobbler	½ cup	3
blueberry cobbler	½ cup	3
custard	½ cup	2
french pastry	1 (4 oz piece)	5
fruit gelatin	½ cup	4½
apple pie	1 slice (average)	7
apricot pie	1 slice	7
berry pie	1 slice	10
butterscotch pie	1 slice	4
cherry pie	1 slice	10
cream pie	1 slice	4
lemon pie	1 slice	7
mince meat pie	1 slice	4
peach pie	1 slice	7
prune pie	1 slice	6
pumpkin pie	1 slice	5
rhubarb pie	1 slice	4
banana pudding	½ cup	2
bread pudding	½ cup	1½
chocolate pudding	½ cup	4
cornstarch pudding	½ cup	2½
date pudding	½ cup	7
fig pudding	½ cup	7
Grapenut pudding	½ cup	2
plum pudding	½ cup	4
rice pudding	½ cup	5
tapioca pudding	½ cup	3
berry tart	1 cup	10
blancmange	½ cup	5

How to improve your nutrition

Food Item	Size Portion	Approximate Sugar Content in Teapsoonful of Granulated Sugar
brown Betty	½ cup	3
plain pastry	1 (4 oz piece)	3
sherbet	½ cup	9

Syrups, Sugars and Icings

brown sugar	1 T	3*
chocolate icing	1 oz	5
chocolate sauce	1 T	3½
corn syrup	1 T	3*
granulated sugar	1 T	3*
honey	1 T	3*
Karo syrup	1 T	3*
maple syrup	1 T	5*
molasses	1 T	3½*
white icing	1 oz	5*

*actual sugar content

Guidelines for nutritional health

- Eat food slowly, chew it well and choose smaller amounts.
- Light snacks between meals and before bed are better than big meals.
- Avoid "instant" foods and products with chemical additives, colorings or compounds which may cause allergies.
- Be careful preparing foods: use polyunsaturated vegetable oils for frying and minimize consumption of fried foods.
- For maximum benefit, quick-steam vegetables, or prepare in a wok.
- Enhance the nutritive value of foods by imaginatively and liberally adding brewer's yeast, wheat germ, lecithin and bone meal in the preparation.
- Take medication only on the advice of a physician.
- Follow a program of regular exercise.

Problems with sugar tolerance are found in those suffering from hypoglycemia (low blood sugar) or diabetes (high blood sugar). If your doctor has told you that you have hypoglycemia, the following program is suggested:

A balanced program for hypoglycemia or low blood sugar

This program is offered to the reader as a suggestion of the author's only. Check with a physician for hypoglycemia tests and symptoms.

Breakfast (the most important meal of the day)

Any two proteins. Examples: natural cheese, eggs, fish, meat, poultry, cottage cheese.

> Fresh fruits
> Herb teas or milk
> Whole-grain bread, optional, or
> Protein drink

Recipe for Hypoglycemic's Protein Drink

1 tsp. lecithin granules	1 tsp. nutritional yeast
drop niacin	1 tsp. acidophilus
1 tsp. vitamin C powder	1 tbs. milk and egg protein
1 tsp. vegetable oil	powder

Combine with 8 to 12 ounces milk, fruit or vegetable juice or water in a blender. Blend for one minute at high speed. Drink 2 ounces or 4 tablespoons every two hours. The protein drink constitutes a complete meal.

Every two hours have either:

(1) Two ounces protein drink and digestive aid if needed, plus 250 mg pantothenic acid, or

(2) Small portion of any type of protein and digestive aid, and

(3) Small portion of any type low carbohydrate vegetable, raw or steamed, and

(4) Small portion of fruit once daily if well-tolerated, or

(4) Six to twelve one-gram chewable protein

tablets, sweetened with fructose if protein drink or protein foods are not available.

Food supplements for a hypoglycemic:

> 3 acidophilus capsules
> 1 multiple vitamin timed release
> 1 vitamin C 1000 mg timed release
> 1 vitamin E 400 IU dry form (d-alphatoco-pheryl succinate)
> 1 B-complex-50
> 1 chelated mineral tablet
> 1 pantothenic acid 250 mg

Multiple digestive enzymes if necessary. All supplements are taken 2 times daily with breakfast and evening meal.

Important: Drink at least 6 glasses of water daily, one-half hour before or after meals.

Avoid at all costs: white sugar, except fruit sugar, white flour, tobacco, alcohol, regular tea, coffee or cola and other "soft" drinks (diet soft drinks included), processed foods and fried foods.

Do you eat too much salt?
(Sodium Chloride NaCl)

Most people in the United States today are ingesting large amounts of salt without even knowing it.

Most of us know that pretzels, potato chips, and french fries are salty but few of us are aware that many other foods such as pastries, cheeses and packaged cereals also contain considerable amounts of salt.

Up to 25 percent of the American public has hypertension or high blood pressure. There is no doubt in my mind that our excessive ingestion of salt is an important factor contributing to high blood pressure.

Some general rules to remember to decrease your salt intake are:

1. Avoid the use of salt at the table, as well as baking soda, monosodium glutamate (MSG, "Accent") and baking powder in food preparation.
2. Avoid laxatives or other substances containing sodium.
3. Do not drink or cook with water treated by a home water softener, as these appliances add sodium to the water.

If you were on a mild sodium restricted diet you would be allowed 2–3 grams of sodium per day. The average American ingests 5–15 grams (approx. ½ oz.) of salt daily.

Let us look at the following table and see how easy it is to go beyond those limits.

Approximate sodium content of common foods

Item	Amount	Salt (mg)
Pickle, dill	1 lge.	1,928
Frozen turkey three-course dinner (Swanson)	1 (17 oz.)	1,735
Soy sauce	1 Tbsp.	1,320
Pancakes (Hungry Jack Complete)	3 pancakes, 4 in. each	1,150
Chicken noodle soup (Campbell's)	10 oz.	1,050
Tomato soup (Campbell's)	10 oz.	950
Green beans, canned (Del Monte)	1 cup	925
Cheese, pasteurized, processed American (Kraft)	2 oz.	890
Baked red kidney beans (B and M)	1 cup	810
Pizza, frozen (Celeste)	4 oz.	656
Danish cinnamon rolls w/raisins (Pillsbury)	1 serv.	630
Pudding, instant chocolate (Jell-o)	½ cup	486
Bologna (Oscar Mayer)	2 slices	450
Tuna, in oil (Del Monte)	3 oz.	430
Frankfurter, beef (Oscar Mayer)	1	425

The most powerful
natural food supplements _____

In the preceding pages, I have written about vitamin and mineral food supplements and nutrition. Now, in alphabetical order I would like to discuss some of the truly healthy foods that unfortunately most Americans do not eat. Some of them have been known since biblical days, some were discovered just a few decades ago, some are in the news today, and some we have forgotten about entirely.

Acidophilus

Lactobacillus acidophilus or acidophilus, as it is commonly known, is stronger than yogurt in producing beneficial intestinal bacteria. It is available as acidophilus culture, incubated in either soy, milk or yeast bases.

Many doctors prescribe acidophilus in conjunction with oral antibiotic treatment because antibiotics destroy the friendly intestinal flora, causing an overgrowth of the fungus monilia albicans. The fungus can grow in the intestines, vagina, lungs, mouth (thrush), on the fingers, or under the finger or toenails. It usually disappears after a few days of large amounts of acidophilus culture.

Putrefaction in the intestines often causes bad breath that is totally resistant to mouthwash or breath spray. This condition is usually accompanied by foul-smelling flatulence. An intensive course of acidophilus culture usually solves this problem.

Lactose, complex carbohydrates, pectin, and vitamin C plus roughage encourages additional growth of intestinal flora. Friendly bacteria can die within five days unless they are continuously supplied with some form of lactic acid or lactose, such as acidophilus.

Antibiotics are often prescribed for acne and other skin problems. The friendly bacteria used internally are usually effective for healing skin conditions. Check with your doctor and try a crash program of eight ounces of acidophilus culture twice a day. Acidophilus can be taken with juice or in milk or plain. Your skin will get worse the first week, as your body eliminates poisons through the pores. After this period, the skin will begin to clear. After the skin is clear, usually two tablespoons after each meal will keep it that way.

Regular use of acidophilus culture keeps the intestines clean and eliminates constipation.

Alfalfa

Frank Bouer, a biologist, author of *This Business of Eating*, has called alfalfa "the great healer." He discovered that the green leaves of this legume contain eight essential enzymes. Later, Dr. C. A. Jacobson, a food scientist with the U.S. government, confirmed these findings. It also seems to contain sufficient vitamin D, lime and phosphorus to make strong bones and teeth in growing children.

Alfalfa is truly valuable for its vitamin content. It contains 8000 IU of vitamin A for every 100 grams. It is a good source of vitamin B6 and vitamin E. It is extremely rich in vitamin K, which protects against hemorrhaging, and helps the blood to clot properly. Alfalfa contains 20,000 to 40,000 units of vitamin K for every 100 grams.

Alfalfa has been used by doctors in treating stomach ailments, gas pains, ulcerous conditions and poor appetite. Alfalfa seems to be useful in stomach ailments because it contains vitamin U. Dr. Garnett of Stanford University stated that vitamin U has great possibilities as an aid for peptic ulcers. Interestingly vitamin U is also found in raw cabbage. Many nutritionists recommend drinking raw cabbage juice as an aid in treating peptic ulcers.

Other uses of alfalfa are its natural diuretic properties (promotes the excretion of urine) and as a natural laxative.

In her book *Feel Like a Million*, Cathryn Elwood, a qualified nutritionist writing about arthritis, stated, "alfalfa, especially the tablets, and lots of them, have seemed to work miracles. Our family doctor has told me of a half dozen patients who have been taking 18 tablets (6, 3 times a day). He says their hands have become more flexible and free from pain." It is not difficult to see why nutritionists call alfalfa "the great healer."

Bee pollen

Throughout the ages, man has valued and made use of bee pollen as a health food and healing agent. Pollen is mentioned in the Bible, Koran and Talmud. Famous and learned men of old, such as the physician Hippocrates, the naturalist Pliny, and the poet Virgil, firmly believed that bee pollen had a most important role to play in making sure of good health and protecting against the many problems associated with old age.

Bee pollen contains all of the eight essential amino acids in varying amounts that fluctuate between five and seven times the amino acids in equal weights of traditional high protein foods. Pollen also contains vitamins A, D, E, K, C and bioflavonoids, as well as the complete B complex, especially pantothenic acid and niacin. This may be the reason why research has shown that pollen puts up a powerful defense against stress as *Prevention* magazine stated in a recent article.

Dr. Peter Hernuss and six colleagues at the University of Vienna's Women's Clinic conducted a study involving twenty five women with inoperable uterine cancer. During the course of radiotherapy, fifteen of the women received a supplement of bee pollen; the other ten served as a control group and were subjected to radiation alone. The pollen was administered three times daily in 20-gram doses. The women receiving the pollen supplement were able to tolerate the radiation stress much better.

In addition to all this goodness, twenty-seven mineral salts and bioelements have been found in bee pollen, including calcium, copper, iron, magnesium, manganese, phosphorus, potassium, silicon, sodium and sulfur.

Dr. Emil Chauvin announced to the French Academy of Science that results of his intensive studies using bee pollen showed that pollen produced an all-around improvement in general health and increased the red blood corpuscles and hemoglobins in anemic patients. He also found it beneficial in cases of chronic prostatitis, constipation, flatulence and infections of the colon, especially diarrhea. Dr. Chauvin also discovered that pollen contains an antibiotic which regulates the intestines by destroying or weakening harmful bacteria and at the same time promoting the growth of friendly bacteria. Bee pollen therapy builds up strength and energy in tired bodies.

Athletes use bee pollen

Finland's Lasse Viren, the 1972 and again 1976 Olympic Gold Medal Distance Champion at 5000 and 10,000 meters, takes 6 to 10 bee pollen supplements a day during training, and from 4 to 6 daily during competition. America's gold medal relay runner, Steve Riddick, credits pollen supplements for better performances.

Bee pollen should be taken fifteen to twenty minutes before a meal, preferably breakfast, when the stomach is completely empty. It may be taken by persons of all ages; in fact, the older the person the more beneficial it may be.

Bran

Current newspaper and magazine articles, and an article in the August 1974 *Journal of the American Medical Association* written by three prominent English physicians, Drs. Burkitt, Walker and Painter, have brought a new concept to preventive medicine, which is really very old.

Is there a correlation between a long-term dietary intake of low fiber refined foods, such as white flour and sugar, and illnesses such as: benign and malignant tumors of the colon and rectum, appendicitis, hemorrhoids, constipation, diverticulosis, gallstones, hiatus hernia and coronary artery diseases?

A research team headed by Dr. Burkitt has found that heart disease, blood clots and obesity are relatively unknown among black Africans outside of cities.

These blacks subsist largely on hand-ground flour and unmilled bran, which permit the digestive process to function completely, removing dangerous substances and synthesizing vital biochemicals.

Many of us in western civilization would live longer, conclude the three physicians, and be a great deal healthier if we ate coarser diets that would send more indigestible dietary fiber through our digestive tracts.

The doctors recommend that we eat breads made of 100 percent whole grains and that we add unprocessed bran to our diets. Bran can be mixed into our regular breakfast cereals. We should try to avoid such foods as canned fruits in favor of raw fruit with the skin or peel.

Bran has little or no food value. We do not digest and absorb it. As it passes through our digestive tract, it accumulates liquid and swells up, providing a good amount of soft bulk that speeds bowel movements.

Bran and gallstones

Report from D. E. W. Pomare, of the Bristol Royal Infirmary, states that extra bran in the diet may help prevent or treat gallstones.

When patients with radiographically-detected gallstones were fed additional bran every day (as much as they could tolerate) in a short-time study, the cholesterol saturation of the bile was significantly lowered, Dr. Pomare told the Canadian Society for Clinical Investigation's Annual Meeting in Winnipeg, Canada (*Internal Medicine News*, March 1, 1975). Cholesterol is the chief constituent of most gallstones.

Dr. Pomare recommends completely unprocessed bran. The larger particle size of unprocessed bran is believed more effective than the smaller particles found in packaged dry cereals, he said.

Dr. Pomare suspects that long-term treatment using an unprocessed bran, might possibly reduce the size of existing gallstones.

Chlorophyll

**Chlorophyll possesses an "antibacterial" action.
It is a wound-healing agent.
New research suggests chlorophyll to be an "antioxidant"
type of substance.**

G. W. Rapp, in the *American Journal of Pharmacy* 121:267, showed chlorophyll to be the most remarkable of all plant products. It has been reported to possess positive antibacterial action.

B. Gruskin, in the *American Journal of Surgery* 49:49–55, stated chlorophyll acts as a direct stimulant to the growth of new tissue while simultaneously reducing the hazard of bacterial contamination, thus acting as a wound-healing agent.

Since the early 1950s chlorophyll has been almost completely forgotten. Now new research is showing that this fascinating substance found in most plants, but not animals, could be an essential anticancer agent.

Chiu-nan lai, in an article entitled "Chlorophyll: The active factor in wheat sprout extract inhibiting the metabolic activation of carcinogens in vitro," tells us that this fundamental green plant substance is the major active factor in wheat sprouts which causes the inhibition of mutagenic (mutation) effects of carcinogens (cancer producing agents).

Wheat grass juice, a popular item in health food stores, shows a similar activity to chlorophyll.

In 1940 chlorophyll was reported by Gruskin to be clinically useful for treating infections and suppurative (pus forming) diseases. He stated, "chlorophyll has never been shown to be toxic in therapeutic doses and its potential as a nontoxic chemo preventative agent appears promising."

Considering this new and old research, it seems to this author that chlorophyll from green vegetables or supplements is a wise dietary component.

Garlic

Can it lower the blood pressure?
Does it have an antibiotic effect?
Is it valuable in treating heart disease?
Why do the Russians call it "Russian penicillin"?
Does it lower blood cholesterol?
Does it clear the blood stream of excess glucose?

Experts from all over the world seem to substantiate these claims. Here are the facts:

Nutritionally speaking, garlic contains potassium and phosphorus, plus a significant amount of B and C vitamins, as well as calcium and protein. In Europe, garlic is respected as a valuable medicine; in America it is ignored. Many medical authorities agree that garlic does reduce high blood pressure. The two theories on its mechanism of action are:

(1) Since garlic is an effective microorganism fighter, it possibly neutralizes the poisonous substances

in the intestines, which results in lowered blood pressure.

(2) Some doctors believe it acts as a vasodilator (i.e., it dilates the blood vessels), thus lowering blood pressure.

F. G. Piotrousky of the University of Vienna found the blood pressure was effectively lowered in 40 percent of his hypertensive patients after they were given garlic.

In *The Lancet*, the journal of the British Medical Association, three Indian physicians revealed that garlic helped in cleansing the blood of excess glucose. It is common knowledge that blood sugar is as important as cholesterol and probably more important in the causation of arteriosclerosis and heart attacks.

Dr. N. Y. Spivak, writing in the Russian journal *Antibiolki,* September 1963, demonstrated garlic's antibacterial properties. Experiments have shown that garlic oil in water quickly alleviated grippe, sore throat and runny nose in patients.

The best way to take garlic is in the form of perles. These capsules contain the valuable garlic oils and leave no after-odor on the breath, because they do not dissolve in the stomach, but in the lower digestive tract. Garlic tablets with parsley (which contains natural chlorophyll) are also available.

It is still difficult to separate fact from fable regarding garlic. The exact value of garlic has not been explored and cannot be defined at present.

Kelp

Kelp contains twenty-three minerals and elements which range as follows:

Iodine	0.15–0.20%	Magnesium	0.76%
Calcium	1.20%	Sulfur	0.93%
Phosphorus	0.30%	Chlorine	12.21%
Iron	0.10%	Copper	0.0008%
Sodium	3.14%	Zinc	0.0003%
Potassium	0.63%	Manganese	0.0008%

Kelp has traces of barium, boron, chromium, lithium, nickel, silver, titanium, vanadium, aluminum, strontium and silicon.

Vitamins present in kelp are: vitamin B2, niacin, choline and carotin. Algenic acid is also present.

This remarkable food contains more vitamins and minerals than any other substance. All these nutrients have been assimilated by the growing plant.

Homeopathic physicians use kelp for obesity, goiter, poor digestion, flatulence and obstinate constipation.

In recent years, the Crenshaw diet of kelp, lecithin, vinegar and B6 has been a popular reducing diet.

Kelp, because of its natural iodine content, acts on the thyroid gland to normalize it. Therefore, thin people with thyroid trouble would gain weight by using kelp and obese people with thyroid trouble would lose weight.

To show you how important the thyroid gland is to human metabolism, here is a list of the thyroid functions:

1. secretes thyroxin
2. controls and regulates metabolism
3. vitalizes every cell of the body and enables them to respond to sympathetic stimulation
4. assists in control of tissue differentiation
5. increases the power and rate of the heart function
6. controls coagulation time for blood clotting
7. increases urea and fluid secretion
8. stimulates and brightens the mind
9. controls and regulates the body fat
10. controls intestinal activity
11. aids the function of the pancreas
12. helps to harmonize the activity of the suprarenal glands
13. has a regulating influence on the ovaries and testicles
14. works in cooperation with the parathyroids, thereby regulating the action of mineral salts in the system, especially of calcium
15. acts in conjunction with the pituitary gland.

Lecithin

Lecithin (pronounced less-i-thin) is found in every cell or organ in the body. It is also necessary to every cell and organ. Theoretically, by eating it in sufficient amounts, you can help rebuild those cells or organs which need it. Once they are repaired, the lecithin helps to maintain their health. To date, there is a mounting accumulation of scientific studies which suggest some of the diverse benefits of lecithin.

Lecithin has been found to reduce the cholesterol level in the blood in some individuals.

It helps dissolve the plaques in the arteries, in some cases.

It also has been noted as of value to eliminate the yellow or yellow-brown plaque on the skin or around the eyes caused by fatty deposits.

Lecithin helps lower the blood pressure in some people.

It produces greater alertness in elderly people.

It increases the gamma globulin in the blood which helps fight infection.

Lecithin benefits certain skin disturbances. These include eczema, acne, and psoriasis.

It fills out and softens aging skin where dryness, paper-thinness and shriveling occur.

It prevents a drawn look during reducing.

Twenty-five years ago, lecithin was used in Germany as a restorative of sexual powers, for glandular exhaustion, as well as for nervous and mental disorders. Seminal fluid is rich in lecithin. Because of its loss from the body, men's need for it may be especially great.

Lecithin is also used in re-distributing weight, by shifting it from areas of the body where it is unwanted to portions where it is needed.

Lecithin helps in the assimilation of vitamin A and E.

It lengthens the lives of animals, producing glossier coats, and greater alertness.

Lecithin, with the additional help of vitamin E, has been found to lower the requirements of insulin in diabetics, in some cases.

Liver

has an anti-anemia factor
has a growth factor
has an energy metabolism factor which resists muscular fatigue
has an anti-estrogen factor

Liver is by far the nearest perfect food, but if you do not like liver, or don't eat it frequently, you are in luck. A perfect substitute is desiccated liver, which is available in tablet or powder form.

The liver is the detoxifying organ of the body, constantly on guard to protect us against poisons. An article appearing in *The Journal of Nutrition*, March 1954, reports that liver, raw or dried, in our diets has been found to be extremely effective against the effects of massive doses of strychnine, sulfanilamide, cortisone, acetate and barbiturates. The protective factor of liver is that it is insoluble in water.

Benjamin H. Ershoff, of the University of Southern California, conducted a well-publicized test with desiccated liver and drug overdose. In his test, Ershoff used desiccated liver, milk protein and the complete B complex of vitamins to determine which would protect his lab animals from overdoses of a drug (Thiouracil), which interferes with the workings of the thyroid gland. Dr. Ershoff deliberately gave his rats huge doses of Thiouracil to see what it would take to protect them against the lethal effects of this poisoning. He found that there was certainly something in desiccated liver that protected the animals against the effects of the drug. The substance was not present in the milk protein or all of the known B vitamins. Desiccated liver not only contains high amounts of iron, but sufficient amounts of the B vitamins so that the body will properly utilize the iron. It includes the whole range of B vitamins, such as vitamins B2, niacin, B12, plus other B factors natural to liver. An additional plus is the whopping 60 percent protein count provided by six tablets.

Papaya, the "magic melon"

prevents your stomach from being queasy
helps digestion
digests 2,230 times its own weight of starch
tenderizes meat

In today's hurried world, we grab, gorge and over-indulge. Unfortunately, our stomachs were not made to take that kind of abuse. What is the usual remedy we run for? You guessed it: antacids that fizzle and sizzle like seltzer and taste like chalk. We down chemicals disguised as candy or mints, or we swallow chalky liquids. There is a natural way to counteract overindulgence. That remedy is nature's own papaya. Papaya enzyme tablets, available in delicious chewable tablet form, can actually digest 2,230 times their weight of starch.

How can papaya do this? Simple. It contains the natural enzymes papain and prolase. These two enzymes assist in protein digestion and combine with mylase, a potent starch digestive enzyme. The best way to take your papaya enzyme tablet is after each meal. Papain is the chief ingredient in meat tenderizers that work on fowl, fish and beef before reaching your stomach.

The U.S. Department of Agriculture notes that "papaya contains peculiar and valuable digestive properties which make it of great value in the diet."

Pectin

Does it lower cholesterol?

Research conducted by Dr. Hans Fisher, Chairman of the Department of Nutrition at Rutgers University, clearly shows that pectin "limits the amount of cholesterol the body can absorb." Dr. Fisher and his associates were quoted as saying that pectin, which is a natural carbohydrate found in fruits and vegetables, "offers partial protection" against the dangerous health problems associated with elevated cholesterol.

In the Rutgers University research teams' work, published in the March 1975 issue of *Nutrition Reports International*, once again pectin showed its ability to lower serum cholesterol levels in various animals. Dr. Fisher reported that college students taking 10 grams of pectin per day for three weeks experienced roughly a 20 percent reduction in average cholesterol levels.

A. S. Truswell and Ruth M. Kay of Queen Elizabeth College's Nutrition Department in London, gave 15 grams of citrus pectin daily in divided doses to three subjects. All showed reduction in cholesterol levels averaging 15 percent. (Reported in *The Lancet*, British Medical Association Journal, April 19, 1975.)

Ten to 15 grams of pectin a day represents about three to six whole apples. Fortunately, pectin is available in concentrated form in tablets. The old adage of "an apple a day" seems more true today than ever before.

Yeast—nature's wonder food

helps prevent heart trouble (with wheat germ)
helps dissolve gallstones
helps reverse gout
helps the aches and stabbing pains of neuritis
helps cancer patients subjected to heavy radiation: (Given yeast daily, some patients did not suffer from the anemia and vomiting which occurred in patients not protected by yeast.)

Yeast is an excellent source of protein and a superior source of the B-complex vitamins. It is one of the richest providers of organic iron as well as most other minerals and trace minerals and amino acids. It stimulates energy and relieves fatigue, constipation, nervousness and indigestion. It is also a perfect reducing food.

Adelle Davis said that yeast helps lower cholesterol (when combined with lecithin), corrects cirrhosis of the liver by rejuvenating the liver, and clears eczema (also acne).

There are various sources of yeast:

Brewer's yeast (from hops, a by-product of beer), sometimes called nutritional yeast

Torula yeast grown on wood pulp used in the manufacture of paper, or from blackstrap molasses

Whey, by-product of milk and cheese
(best tasting and most potent)

Liquid yeast from Switzerland and Germany, fed on herbs, honey malt and or-
anges or grapefruit.

Avoid live baker's yeast. Live yeast cells are vitamin robbers, especially of B vitamins in the intestines. In nutritional yeast, these live cells are heat
killed, and thus are prevented from stealing B vitamins from your body. Yeast has all the major B
vitamins except B12, which can be especially bred
into it; yeast contains 16 amino acids, 14 or more
minerals, and 17 vitamins (except for A, E and C).
Yeast can be considered a whole food. Because
yeast, like other protein food, is high in phosphorus,
it is advisable when taking it to add extra calcium
to the diet. Phosphorus a co-worker of calcium, can
take calcium out of the body with it, leaving a calcium deficiency. The remedy is simple: take extra
calcium (calcium lactate assimilates well in the
body). B complex should be taken with yeast to be
more effective. Together they work like a power-
house.

Yeast can be stirred into liquid, juice or water and
taken between meals. Many people who feel fa-
tigued take a tablespoon or more in liquid and feel
a return of energy within minutes and the good effects last for several hours. Yeast can be used as a
reducing food. Stir into liquid and drink it just be-

fore a meal, and it takes the edge off a large appetite and saves eating too many calories.

(*Let's Eat Right to Keep Fit*, by Adelle Davis. *Nutrition Almanac*, Nutrition Search Inc. *Secrets of Health and Beauty*, by Linda Clark.)

Yucca extract tablets

Can yucca help arthritis?

This desert plant is a genus of trees and shrubs belonging to the liliaceae family. The Joshua Tree is a yucca reaching an average height of twenty to thirty feet. Other yucca reach six to eighteen feet in height. The primitive Indians used yucca for many purposes and revered it almost as a god—or at least a special, god-given plant which guaranteed their health and survival.

Dr. John W. Yale, Ph.D., a botanical biochemist, extracted the steroid saponin from the yucca plant. Dr. Yale approached the National Arthritis Medical Clinic in Desert Hot Springs, California, to see if there was any interest in a yucca extract tablet in the treatment of arthritis. In 1973, a one-year study was begun. Briefly, the results showed the yucca steroid saponin proved favorably in a sufficient percentage of cases to justify its use in the overall management of arthritis. It also proved to be non-toxic. Dosage varied from 2 to 8 tablets daily, with an average of 4 tablets daily. The tablets were taken before, during and after meals with no resulting problems. They caused no gastro-intestinal tract irritation.

Of the 165 patients tested, over 60 percent felt

less pain, stiffness and swelling, the three major complaints of arthritis. The rest felt no change. The effects were felt from four days to three months later.

The roles of protein, amino acids, lipotropics and enzymes in nutrition———

Protein

supplies the body with energy
is necessary for growth in children
is necessary for adults to maintain their body structure.

Every cell in your body contains protein.

Protein is the basic nutrient capable of building, repairing, and maintaining all the body tissues. Protein is the master builder of the human body. It is the most complex substance known to man. Protein contains nitrogen and sulfur which break up or "oxidize" to obtain energy.

Foods highest in protein are:

1. meat, fish
2. eggs
3. cheese made from milk
4. lentils, soybeans
5. Brazil nuts
6. oats, sweet potatoes (high quality protein)

Can nucleic acid slow, halt or reverse the aging process?

DNA (Deoxyribonucleic acid) is a protein. Every cell nucleus contains DNA. Its job is to put together the final products of the body. For example, if you need a liver protein replacement, DNA will send out a message to that effect. The amino acids are gathered in the proper sequence as a chain, or spiral, or rod, or sphere, and the new protein is then shipped to wherever it is needed.

Benjamin S. Frank, M.D., in his book *Nucleic Acid Therapy in Aging and Degenerative Disease* (Psychological Library, New York, 1969, revised 1974), describes the formulations by which he believes he has been able to push back the aging process. His approach is directed to the nucleus of the cell.

Further research has revealed that the nucleic acids deoxyribonucleic acid (DNA) and ribonucleic acid (RNA) are the cellular components which control heredity and the subsequent ability of the body to keep reproducing its inherited patterns. These strands of acid within the cell nucleus govern all life processes in health and disease.

Dr. Frank's work with DNA and RNA demonstrates the importance of these substances, not only to longer life free of disease, but to the wonderful quality of being young as long as you live.

What is it that permits the skin on the back of an aged hand to become shiny, wrinkled, spotted and brittle? The cells which contain the blueprint for the formation of that hand are tired and worn, and no longer able to maintain the pattern they inherited. In Dr. Frank's opinion the problem of maintaining youthfulness is to find ways to help the body's DNA and RNA renew themselves and keep their patterns of genetic information as clean and fresh as a new etching. Dr. Frank considers the solution is to supply the body from external sources with enough viable nucleic acids and with the other nutrients these nucleic acids require to be properly metabolized.

The results of Dr. Frank's experimental studies provide strong evidence that RNA does indeed visibly reverse aging, especially when given along with other metabolites such as B-complex and other vitamins and minerals.

Dr. Frank found that the needed doses of RNA varied from 30 milligrams to 300 milligrams daily, plus B-complex factors in the form of therapeutic vitamin and mineral tablets. The most immediate effect was an increase in energy and wellbeing, even in lower dosage. In higher dosage, these effects were observed more rapidly, sometimes in two or three days. The facial skin became healthier, rosier and smoother. After one or two months of treatment, there not only was an increase in smoothness and color of the skin, but lines and wrinkles began to diminish.

Amino acids

There are twenty-two components of protein called amino acids. Only fourteen amino acids are produced in the body; the other eight must be supplied from food intake.

Y-BUTYRIC AMINO ACID
One of the best known substances that transmit nerve impulses to the brain.

GLYCINE
Serves as a stimulant to the brain. It also aids in healing of swollen and infected prostate.

GLUTAMIC ACID
May serve as a brain stimulant. It provides Y-butyric amino acid.

TYROSINE
Acts in regulation of emotional behavior. Important in eventual synthesis of thyroxine thus aiding in prevention of hypothyroidism. It also yields L-dopa, which has a side effect of increasing sexuality.

*THREONINE
Deficiency results in negative hydrogen balance in the body.

*LEUCINE
It is found to be lacking in alcoholics and drug addicts, as are three other amino acids, L-glutamine, A-amino-n-butyric acid, and citruline.

ARGININE
Increases the sperm content in the male.

*PHENYLALANINE
It cannot be metabolized if a person is deficient in vitamin C. It is a stimulant which sends impulses to the brain, acts as an antidepressant and can raise blood pressure.

*TRYPTOPHAN

It provides niacin which prevents pellagra and mental deficiency. It regulates sleep. Deficiency causes insomnia. It is useful as a relaxant as well.

A natural help for insomnia

Tests show that tryptophan may dramatically reduce the time it takes the average insomniac to fall asleep. The tests were reported at the Maryland Psychiatric Research Center at a symposium on sleep held at Johns Hopkins University.

If the pills prove out in further trials, they may go a long way toward solving two problems at once: the individual insomniac's trouble in sleeping, and the growing menace of barbiturate addiction.

Dr. Althea Wagman who, along with Dr. Clinton C. Brown is conducting the research says, "Tryptophan is a natural part of a person's physical makeup. The body doesn't have to change any function to make use of tryptophan, as it does to make use of barbiturates. That means there's no danger of tryptophan addiction or overdose."

Dr. Brown adds, "Furthermore, the sleep that is induced by tryptophan is a natural sleep, not the 'knock-out' unconsciousness induced by barbiturates."

Tryptophan may keep alcoholics dry

A diet supplement of tryptophan may help alcoholics stay dry by relieving some of the symptoms of alcohol-related body chemistry disorders, the Veterans Administration research indicates.

Given in larger concentrations than occur in a normal diet, tryptophan helps alcoholics achieve normal sleeping patterns because it reduces or normalizes the fragmentation of dreaming (REM) sleep in alcoholic patients.

The finding is important because serotonin, a natural tranquilizer substance in the brain, has been shown to be reduced in alcoholism.

*Isoleucine
Needed in hemoglobin formation

Cystine and *Methionine
Natural chelating agents for heavy metals. They aid in producing beautiful skin. Methionine can be substituted for choline which aids in reducing liver fat (lipotropic agent) and protects the kidneys. It also builds new body tissue. A deficiency of methionine may lead to fatty degeneration and cirrhosis of the liver.

Methionine can be found in meat, eggs, fish, milk and cheese.

Histidine
Precursor of histamine. It keeps people from biting their nails. Dilates blood vessels.

*Lysine
Deficiency may cause nausea, dizziness and anemia.

L-lysine monohydrochloride builds new body tissue and also such vital substances as antibodies, hormones, enzymes and body cells.

Lysine is found in meat, eggs, fish, milk and cheese. It is useful against cold sores or fever blis-

---

*Essential amino acids (cannot be made by the body).

ters in 500 mg to 3 gram dosage. All amino acids should be taken in between meals with juice or water—not with protein.

VALINE

Deficiency results in negative hydrogen balance in the body.

Four important functions of lipotropics
(methionine—choline—inositol—betaine)

1. They increase production of lecithin by the liver
This helps to keep cholesterol more soluble, thereby lessening cholesterol deposits in blood vessels and also lessening the chances of gallstone formation. (Gallstones usually have a large percentage of cholesterol deposits.)

2. They prevent accumulation of fats in the liver
Fatty liver is probably the main reason for sluggish liver function. Methionine seems to act as a catalyst for choline and inositol, speeding up their function.

3. They detoxify the liver
Methionine and choline detoxify amines which are by-products of protein metabolism. This is especially important for persons on a high-protein diet.

4. They increase resistance to disease
Lipotropics help to increase resistance to disease by bolstering the thymus gland in carrying out its anti-disease function in three ways:

- by stimulating the production of antibodies
- by stimulating the growth and action of phagocytes, which surround and gobble up invading viruses and microbes
- by recognizing and destroying foreign and abnormal tissue.

Enzymes

Enzymes are complex proteins necessary for the digestion of food. They release valuable vitamins, minerals and amino acids which keep us alive and healthy. Enzymes are catalysts, i.e., they have the power to cause an internal action without changing or destroying themselves in the process. Each enzyme acts upon a specific food; one cannot substitute for the other. A shortage or deficiency, or even the absence of one single enzyme, can make all the difference between health and sickness.

Because enzymes are destroyed under certain conditions of heat, uncooked or unprocessed fruits, vegetables, eggs, meats and fish, are excellent sources.

Pepsin is a vital digestive enzyme which breaks up the proteins of ingested food, splitting them into usable amino acids. Without pepsin, protein could not be used to build healthy skin, strong skeletal structure, rich blood supply and strong muscles.

Renin is a digestive enzyme which causes coagulation of milk, changing its protein, casein, into a usable form in the body. Renin releases the valuable minerals from milk—calcium, phosphorus, potassium and iron which are used by the body to stabilize the water balance, strengthen the nervous system and produce strong teeth and bones.

Lipase splits fat, which is then utilized to nourish the skin cells, protect the body against bruises and blows, and ward off the entrance of infectious virus cells and allergic conditions.

Hydrochloric acid in the stomach works on tough foods such as fibrous meats, vegetables and poultry.

Other roles in nutrition

A deficiency of HCl in the stomach can cause improper digestion, as well as loss of valuable vitamins and minerals. Betaine HCl and glutamic acid HCl are the best forms of commercially available hydrochloric acid.

Recently, I attended a lecture by Dr. Alan Nittler, author of *A New Breed of Doctor,* which rearoused my interest in hydrochloric acid. He stated emphatically that everyone over the age of 40 should be using HCl.

After watching all those television commercials, you are probably saying to yourself that you don't need any more acid since you have an overacid problem of heartburn, and are taking an antacid, such as Maalox, Mylanta, Digel, Tums, Rolaids or Alka-Seltzer. According to Linda Clark in *Know Your Nutrition,* you may have exactly the opposite problem. HCl is a digestive acid secreted in normal stomachs. It digests protein, calcium, and iron. Without HCl, you can be subject to pernicious anemia, gastric carcinoma, congenital achlorhydria and allergy. Since the symptoms of too little acid are just the same as too much acid, the taking of antacids could be the worst possible thing to do.

Dr. Hugh Tuckey stated that the trial and error method is the best way to discover whether you need HCl supplementation or not. He suggests taking an HCl tablet with betaine plus pepsin after a protein meal. If that "lump feeling" or gas remains you may have too much acid, which is rare indeed. To overcome this burning sensation, drink a glass of water, which flushes away the excess HCl.

"The rat race," stress, tension, anger and worry before eating can all cause a lack of HCl. Deficiencies of some vitamins (B complex primarily) and minerals can also cause a lack of HCl.

Most of us eat too quickly and do not allow our systems to digest food correctly. People with flatulence (gas) can cause the condition themselves by gulping down food and actually inhaling air too quickly.

To sum up, if I can borrow an old television commercial slogan, "Try HCl, you'll like it."

Modern maladies _____

Excess Cholesterol

Basically, cholesterol is a fat-like substance used in many of the body's chemical processes. To maintain good health, our bodies require a certain amount of cholesterol. What we don't need is an elevated serum cholesterol which, unfortunately, too many of us have. The *Merck Manual*, 12th edition, states, "The desirable level of serum cholesterol (cholesterol in the blood) is 150 to 200 mg/100 ml; values greater than 250 mg/100 ml are abnormal." Only a physician can determine your cholesterol level.

WHAT DOES CHOLESTEROL DO?
Excess cholesterol that cannot be utilized by the body enters your blood stream. Cholesterol deposits can build up on the coronary arteries. Slowly but steadily, year after year, this build up continues.

The outcome is artery walls thickened by plaque-like deposits. Less blood and oxygen can be delivered to the heart muscle. Thus the heart has to work harder. A heart attack may occur if the blockage in the artery becomes severe enough.

What Changes in Your Diet Are Needed To Reduce Cholesterol?

As much as possible, try to reduce your intake of foods high in cholesterol or containing "saturated fats"—these fats seem to contribute most to high cholesterol levels. Your diet should be rich in "polyunsaturated fats."

Why Are Polyunsaturated Foods Important?

Polyunsaturates help to lower cholesterol levels. The mechanism action is unknown but it seems that they may help your body to reduce cholesterol deposits that are already formed. Many physicians recommend the following steps to reduce your risk of a heart attack:

1. Replace saturated fats with polyunsaturated fats whenever possible
2. Keep your weight at normal levels
3. Stop smoking
4. Avoid stress
5. Exercise regularly
6. Have regular checkups.

Heart disease (see pp. 64, 68, 75)

Drinking and Smoking are Dangerous to Your Health

People who drink and smoke are twice as prone to dying from cancer as those who do not.

Here are some recent findings:

A two-year study by James E. Enstrom, a public health scientist at the University of California at Los Angeles (UCLA), shows that the death rate from cancer among Mormons and Seventh-Day Adventists is about half that of the general U.S. population. Mormons and Seventh-Day Adventists who observe the rules of their faiths neither smoke nor drink.

VITAMINS FOR SMOKERS AND DRINKERS

For persons with bad drinking and smoking habits, Dr. Herbert Sprince of Jefferson Medical College in Philadelphia has some encouraging news.

Research by Dr. Sprince and associates shows that combined dosage of vitamin B1 (thiamin, one of the B-complex vitamins), vitamin C and cysteine (an amino acid) protects rats against normal lethal doses of acetaldehyde. This chemical (acetaldehyde) is found in tobacco smoke and is also the first by-product formed in the body after a drink of alcohol.

Dr. Sprince emphasizes that there is a long way to go before his findings are incorporated into treatment for humans. Nevertheless, he says, "The public should be informed. Even though the work was done with rats, there's strong feeling that this may be helpful in human therapy."

DRINKING INCLUDES BEER AND WINE

Chronic heavy consumption of alcohol, including

beer and wine, can interfere with the body's utilization of vitamins B1 (thiamin), B6 (pyridoxine) and folic acid. Also, heavy drinking is frequently accompanied by poor eating habits, which compounds the problem by reducing vitamin intake.

Nutrition for special needs_____

Nutrition for travelers

The average American family saves for 50 weeks a year to go on a two-week vacation. A great deal of planning and expense goes into that two- or three-week or even month-long trip. If you are planning a trip to Europe, Mexico or the Orient, a few words about nutrition can give you a more fruitful and healthy experience.

In Europe, a continental breakfast supplies you with rolls, coffee and marmalade. This meal was not designed to promote energy production, nor are late European dinners conducive to early morning appetites. Approximately 20 grams of protein are required per meal, i.e., two eggs, and a glass of milk or a large steak. A continental breakfast gives you two to four grams of protein.

A good multivitamin-mineral supplement with a complete B complex is essential. B vitamins are available in brewer's yeast and liver tablets. Vitamin C is also very important. Five hundred milligram tablets are the most convenient. For travelers on a hectic schedule (if it's Tuesday, this must be Belgium) antistress B complex, high in B vitamins and at least 100 mg of pantothenic acid might come in handy.

In Asian countries where protein is not prominent in the diet, a pep-up protein powder added to your juice in the morning will give you extra energy. If possible, eat yogurt on your vacation. The friendly bacteria can help to prevent dysentery. Yogurt is available in concentrated tablet form also. The yogurt bacteria (lactobacillus acidophilus) breaks milk sugar into lactic acid and discourages the growth of pathogenic organisms. Two or three yogurt tablets a day, seven days before your vacation and during it, give the best results.

Remember, you are paying a lot for your vacation; you might as well enjoy it in the best of health.

Have a great time!

Nutrition for insomnia (see tryptophan, page 83)

Nutrition for healthy skin and hair

HIGH PROTEIN/LOW CARBOHYDRATE DIET

Daily: Fish, chicken, beef, eggs, milk. Some
(55–65 protein at each meal (broiled, baked or
grams) boiled). Fresh vegetables, raw salads, raw sprouts, steamed fresh vegetables (vitamins B, C and E). Fresh fruit after

each meal and during evening. One or two slices whole wheat bread. Eight glasses water (including herbal teas—rose hips, comfrey and golden seal), non-fat milk and non-fat yogurt. Do not use cola drinks, soft drinks, coffee, alcohol, cigarettes or excessive salt.

Supplements

MULTIPLE VITAMIN AND MINERAL COMPLEX
Daily: 1 after breakfast, lunch or dinner. For
(1) skin, eyes, energy and nerve health.

B-COMPLEX 100 MG TIME-RELEASE TABLET
Daily: 1 after breakfast, lunch or dinner. B vi-
(1) tamins essential for skin and energy health. B2 (riboflavin) and B6 (pyriodoxine) reduce facial oiliness and blackhead formation.

DRY A
Daily: 1 after breakfast and 1 after dinner. Aids
(2) in growth and repair of body tissues and maintains soft, smooth, disease-free skin (skin blemishes). Nourishes skin. Builds resistance to all kinds of infections.

1000 mg VITAMIN C WITH ROSE HIPS TIMED RELEASE
Daily: 1 after each meal and 1 at bedtime. Re-
(4) sists and aids in resisting spread of acne infection. Promotes healing of wounds, bruising and scar tissue. Forms collagen and strengthens connective tissues. Aids

in prevention of breakage of capillary veins on face.

DRY E-400 IU

Daily:
(3)

1 after breakfast, 1 after lunch and 1 after dinner. Vitamin E can improve circulation in tiny capillaries on face. It can aid internally in healing of skin and cell formation by replacing the cells on the outer layer of the skin. Vitamin E and C work together to keep blood vessels healthy and less subject to skin disturbances (acne). Use vitamin E oil externally on skin for healing of burns, abrasions and scar tissue.

ZINC

Daily:
(1–3)

1 50 mg (chelated) tablet after each meal. Maintains healthy skin. Aids in growth and repair of injured tissues. Necessary for tissue respiration. Zinc deficiency is a factor in susceptibility to infection. Adding zinc to the diet aids the healing of wounds and infections.

CHOLINE AND INOSITOL

Daily:
1000mg
or 3
tablets

1 after breakfast, lunch and dinner. Also available in the natural source of lecithin granules. Take 2 tablespoons daily if you prefer instead of the 3 tablets of choline and inositol. Helps to emulsify cholesterol (fatty deposits or bumps— acne—under the skin). Essential for a healthy nervous system. Cleanses the

liver and purifies the kidneys, resulting in a clear, smooth, healthy skin.

ACIDOPHILUS

Daily:
6 tbs.

2 tablespoons after each meal or 6 capsules after each meal. Acidophilus has a live, friendly bacteria that clings to the intestinal walls and fights unfriendly bacteria caused by infection, colds, etc. Acidophilus is helpful in fighting the skin eruptions unfriendly bacteria cause and works as an intestinal cleanser.

CHLOROPHYLL

Daily:
3 tsp. or 9 tablets

1 teaspoon after each meal or 3 tablets. Chlorophyll is a wound-healing agent and a direct stimulant to the growth of new tissue, while at the same time reducing the hazard of bacterial contamination. Possesses antibiotic action. Chlorophyll lotion used twice daily is an excellent aid to healing—after washing thoroughly with a soap substitute made from the comfrey plant. Proper nutrition and skin cleanliness, together with adequate rest, exercise, fresh air and sunlight are helpful in the treatment of acne. Do not use makeup if possible; use any cosmetic preparations at a minimum.

Protein drink
(for a healthy, glowing skin)

8 ounces low-fat milk

1 tablespoon yeast powder (B vitamins for skin)
3 tablespoons acidophilus (promotes friendly bacteria)
1 tablespoon granulated lecithin (breaks down bumps or cholesterol under the skin)
2 tablespoons milk and egg protein powder
½ to 1 tablespoon blackstrap molasses (high in minerals and iron) may also be used as a sweetener instead of honey
For flavoring use carob powder, bananas, strawberries, or any fresh fruit
Mix in blender. Add 3–4 ice cubes, if desired.

Protein drink can be taken in place of one meal daily, preferably breakfast.

BE KIND TO YOUR HAIR

Nutrition plays a very important role in having healthy, shiny hair. Poor eating habits and stress can cause hair to fall out.

In Adelle Davis's *Let's Get Well*, she states that increasing your protein intake, particularly liver, wheat germ and nutritional yeast, and supplementing the diet with 1000 mg of inositol (a B vitamin) daily, usually prevents hair loss. The growth of hair is influenced by certain members of the vitamin B family, iron and iodine. A lack of iron, copper, iodine and some of the amino acids also may contribute to a dwindling supply of hair.

Adelle Davis also recommends that three B vitamins—pantothenic acid, folic acid and para-aminobenzoic acid (PABA)—can help restore natural color to gray hair. In male animals massive doses of inositol have caused a regrowth of hair on bald spots.

All three anti-gray B vitamins should be taken together with food and a complete B-complex vitamin.

Vitamins A and E, which work together, are also important for healthy, lustrous hair.

Choline and inositol are available in tablet form. Best natural source is lecithin, which is available in capsules, powder, granules, and liquid.

Iodine is found in fish and kelp tablets.

Iron: Best natural source is liver, wheat germ, yeast and molasses. Organic iron is ferrous gluconate, funerate or peptonate.

Minerals such as silicon and sulfur are necessary for healthy hair.

Finally, frequent scalp massage and a good pH-balanced, protein-enriched shampoo will enhance the beauty of your hair by making it shinier and thicker.

Nutrition for stress and tension

In today's tense world stress can cause diseases such as ulcers, colitis and high blood pressure. In fact, it has been stated that 75 percent of the patients of a general practice physician have some symptoms caused by emotionally induced illness. It is interesting to note that the weakest part of the human anatomy is the gastro-intestinal tract (or the gut).

It has been proven that during times of stress, the body's need for certain nutrients is greatly increased. Increased tension and stress is usually accompanied by inability to sleep, loss or gaining of weight, exhaustion, irritability, depression and loss of emotional control, as well as numerous aches and pains, either small or large.

Pituitary and adrenal hormones are the body's way of counteracting prolonged stress. This is where nutrition begins to play a very significant role. Vitamins E, pantothenic acid and the remainder of the B-complex vitamins are necessary for the proper functioning of the pituitary and adrenal glands. Vitamin C need during stress is increased greatly because it accelerates the rate of cortisone production. Also, vitamin C may be the detoxifying agent the body needs during stress conditions.

There are certain vitamin-like substances called anti-stress factors that we do not as yet know about. These factors are found in wheat germ, yeast, kidney and soy flour. (Interestingly enough, each food is a good source of either vitamin E, B complex or protein.) Therefore, during a stressful period, throw away your candy bars, potato chips and coffee, and reach for milk and protein. All these nutrients should be used in larger amounts: Vitamin C, all the B vitamins plus pantothenic acid, vitamins E, A and D and calcium and magnesium. Calcium is essential for nerve tissue and magnesium is involved with the functioning of the brain and nervous system.

Nutrition for special energy demands
BREAKFAST (The most important meal of the day)
A combination of at least 2 proteins
Examples: natural cheese, eggs, fish, meat, poultry, cottage cheese
Fresh fruit, herb tea or milk
One slice whole grain bread (optional)

Pep-Up Protein Drink

1 tablespoon milk and egg protein powder
1 tablespoon lecithin granules
1 tablespoon acidophilus liquid
1 tablespoon nutritional yeast
1 tablespoon safflower oil (optional)

Blend with 8 ounces milk or juice in blender one minute. 3 ice cubes and fresh fruit can be added for taste and frothiness.

Lunch—*the same as breakfast*

Mid-Afternoon Pick-Up

Small portion of protein or protein drink consisting of 1 to 2 tablespoons of milk and egg protein powder in milk or juice.

Dinner

Chef's salad, any fresh vegetables, hard-boiled eggs, small portion of shrimp, tuna or ham and natural cheese. Herb tea hot or cold, or milk, romaine lettuce, endive, beets, cucumbers, red cabbage, asparagus, green peppers, carrots, celery, tomatoes.
Drink at least 6 glasses of water daily ½ hour before or ½ after meals.

Snacks

Natural peanut butter, yogurt, whole grain bread with safflower margarine.

Avoid

Sugar, except fruit sugar; flour, tobacco, alcohol, regular tea, coffee, soft drinks (including diet), processed foods and fried foods.

Supplements recommended:

with breakfast:

1 high potency multiple vitamin and mineral supplement

2 high potency B with C

1 vitamin E 400 IU

2 multiple chelated minerals

3 acidophilus capsules or 2 tablespoons liquid acidophilus

1 tablespoon lecithin granules or 3-1200 mg lecithin capsules

Options: Nucleic complex, liver, B12, digestive enzymes

with lunch:

2 high potency B with C

1 vitamin E 400 IU

3 acidophilus capsules or 2 tablespoons liquid acidophilus

3 lecithin capsules 1200 mg

Optional: B12, liver tablets, digestive enzymes

with dinner:

2 high potency B with C

1 vitamin E 400 IU

3 acidophilus capsules or 2 tablespoons liquid acidophilus

3 lecithin capsules 19-grain

Optional: Digestive enzymes

Nutrition for athletes

HIGH PROTEIN DIET

Eggs, fish, chicken, beef, cheese, milk, nuts
Some protein at each meal
Fresh vegetables—raw salads and steamed fresh
vegetables
1 or 2 slices whole grain bread
4 glasses milk (including yogurt and kefir)

Do not use sugar; use honey for energy and
sweetening
Do not use frozen or canned foods
Do not use processed foods

Supplements after meals

HIGH POTENCY MULTIPLE VITAMINS
AND MINERALS
Daily: 1 after breakfast—1 after lunch or din-
(2)   ner. After the two largest meals of the
             day for energy, eyes, skin and nerve
             health.

ROSE HIPS—VITAMIN C 1000 mg WITH BIOFLA-
VONOIDS
Daily: 1 after each meal and 1 at bedtime. Heals
(4)   bruises and eases muscle strain. Pre-
             vents sore muscles. Provides resistance
             to colds. Forms collagen in connective
             tissues. Works on adrenal glands when
             under stress, strain and pressure.

CHELATED MINERALS

Daily:
(2)
1 with breakfast and dinner. Aids in muscle growth. Guards against muscle cramps, backache, foot and leg cramps, nervousness. Good for teeth, bones, nerves and skeleton health.

VITAMIN E—400 IU

Daily:
(2)
1 with breakfast and dinner. Retards aging. Contains an anti-clotting factor and increases blood flow to the heart. Maintains muscles and nerves. Increases male potency. Brings oxygen into body and heart and makes the heart a more efficient pump. Aids circulation. Helps endurance and capacity for working out for longer periods without running out of oxygen.

VITAMIN F [unsaturated fatty acids]

Daily:
(2Tb)
2 tablespoons daily. Vitamin F is found in cold pressed oils such as safflower, soy, corn or wheat germ oil. It destroys cholesterol, helps prevent hardening of the arteries and normalized blood pressure. Corrects eczema, psoriasis and other skin problems. Regulates overweight or underweight problems.

DESICCATED LIVER TABLETS

Daily:
(45 to 60)
15 to 20 tablets after each meal. Excellent for building muscles. Builds and repairs tissues and cells. Liver has iron for energy and B12 for building better

blood. Helps stress and disease resistance.

LECITHIN

Daily:
(18)

6 capsules after each meal or 3 tablespoons of granules daily. 1 tablespoon after each meal to emulsify cholesterol because of high protein diet.

WHEAT GERM OIL CAPSULES

Daily:
(9)

3 after each meal. These essential oils aid in endurance and energy in competition. Aids in hormone production. Stimulates glandular activity (adrenal and thyroid glands).

PROTEIN DRINK

Daily:
(2)

After 2 meals for building muscles and weight gain.

2 tablespoons acidophilus (source of good bacteria)

8 ounces milk

3 tablespoons protein powder (builds and repairs tissues)

1 tablespoon yeast powder (B vitamins for energy)

1 tablespoon cold-pressed safflower oil (vitamin F)

1 tablespoon lecithin *granules*

Honey for sweetening, fruit, carob powder, banana

Any concentrate (cherry, etc.) for flavoring

Mix in blender—add 3 to 4 ice cubes if desired.

My basic vitamin-mineral program for beginners _____

1. A complete multiple timed release vitamin with chelated minerals taken one in the morning with or after food and one with your evening meal.
2. A C-complex timed release vitamin with 1000 mg of C plus rose hips and the bioflavonoids plus hesperidin and rutin, taken one in the morning with or after food and one with your evening meal.
3. Vitamin E 400 IU. Taken one with breakfast and one with evening meal.
4. A complete high potency multiple chelated mineral, taken one with breakfast and one with your evening meal.

As you become more sophisticated in nutrition, I would suggest using lecithin capsules or granules, RNA-DNA, SOD, acidophilus and a multiple digestive enzyme.

Drugs can deplete
the body's store of nutrients _____

Today more than ever before, Americans are gulping down drugs (prescription and non-prescription, (or over the counter) in record amounts. All one has to do is watch television one night. Headaches, runny noses, sore throats, constipation, diarrhea, upset stomach, allergies and sinus problems, etc. can all be overcome by downing Drug A or Drug B, on to Drug Z.

What America does not realize is that many of these drugs actually cause depletion of the body's essential vitamins and minerals. A recent scientific study shows that ingredients found in common over-the-counter (OTC) cold, pain and allergic remedies actually lower the blood level of vitamin A in animals. Because vitamin A protects and strengthens the mucous membranes lining the nose, throat and lungs, a deficiency of vitamin A could actually break down these membranes, giving bacteria a cozy home to multiply in. Therefore, the drugs that are supposed to alleviate the cold may be actually prolonging it!

Side effects of drugs are well known. Antihistamines can cause drowsiness, aspirin can cause stomach upset. But what most of us do not know is that they can also cause a nutritional deficiency. Many drugs either stop the absorption of nutrients or interfere with the cell's ability to use them.

Which drugs deplete vitamins and minerals?

ASPIRIN

In 1977 in the U.S.A., 37 million pounds of aspirin were consumed. It is the most common ingredient in many prescription and non-prescription pain relievers, cold remedies, and sinus remedies. A study has shown that even a small amount of aspirin can triple the excretion rate of vitamin C from the body.

Many millions take aspirin to relieve the pain and inflammation of arthritis. What they don't know is that aspirin not only depletes the body of vitamin C, but it also can lead to a deficiency of folic acid, one of the B vitamins. A deficiency of folic acid can lead to anemia, digestive disturbances, graying hair and growth problems.

CORTICOSTEROIDS (Cortisone, Prednisone) belong to another class of drugs used to ease the pain of arthritis. They are also prescribed for skin problems, blood and eye disorders and asthma. Researchers conducted a study of 24 asthmatics using cortisone-type drugs and found the zinc levels were 42 percent lower than in patients not treated with corticosteroids.

A zinc deficiency can lead to loss of taste and smell as well as a loss in sexual desire. Zinc is necessary for male potency and the health of the prostate gland. Zinc also enhances wound healing and is essential for a clear complexion.

THE PILL (oral contraceptive, birth control pill) is a synthetic hormone. It is a powerful drug which convinces a woman's body that she is pregnant. It can also lead to a deficiency of zinc, folic acid, vitamins C, B6 and B12. Deficiency of B12 can lead to a nervous condition. B6 deficiency can cause depression (many women on the pill are depressed).

Women taking oral contraceptives (birth control pills) should take at least 25–30 mg of B6, 4 mg of B12, and 800 mg of folic acid. Vitamin C is depleted by a minimum of 100 mg daily. Low vitamin C levels may account for increased susceptibility to blood-clotting.

BARBITURATES (Phenobarb, Seconal, Nembutal, Butisol) are strong sedatives and hypnotics which are prescribed for insomnia. A study done in the *Postgraduate Medical Journal 1977* reveals that a significant number of people tested who took barbiturates had low calcium levels. A lack of calcium can cause osteoporosis and muscle cramps.

LAXATIVES AND ANTACIDS are routinely prescribed for digestive complaints, constipation or ulcer.

In the June 15, 1975 edition of *Medical World News*, Dr. Herta Spencer found that OTC antacids that contain aluminum (Gelusil, Wingel, Kolantyl, Maalox, Aludrox, Creamalin, Gaviscon, Mylanta, Di-Gel, Rolaids) disturb the calcium and phosphorus metabolism. Phosphorus deficiency, which is very rare (except in antacid users), can cause fatigue, loss of appetite and fragile bones.

MINERAL OIL (a lubricant laxative) prevents absorption of vitamins A and D. Any laxative taken to excess can flush out large amounts of potassium, which can cause heart problems and muscle weakness.

DIURETICS commonly prescribed for high blood pressure, also flush potassium out of the body. And antibiotics can also rob the body of potassium.

I have compiled a list of drugs which induce vitamin deficiencies and the vitamins they deplete. Check it out before you take your next medicine.

I. Drugs Which Induce Vitamin Deficiencies

Three basic mechanisms exist by which drugs induce vitamin deficiencies:
A. Impaired vitamin absorption
B. Impaired vitamin utilization
C. Enhanced vitamin elimination.

A. **IMPAIRMENT OF VITAMIN ABSORPTION**	*Vitamins Depleted*
Glutethimide (Doriden)	folic acid
Cholestyramine (Cuemid, Questran)	A, D, E, K, & B12
Os-Cal-Mone	B6
Mineral Oil	A, D, E, & K
Polysporin, Neo-Sporin, Neomycin, Mycolog, Neo-Cortef, Cortisporin, Lidosporin, Mycifradin	K, B12 & folic acid
Kanamycin (Kantrex)	K & B12
Tetracycline (Achromycin, Sumycin, Tetracyn)	K, calcium, magnesium and iron
Chloramphenical (Chloromycetin)	K
Polymyxin (Aerosporin)	K
Sulfonamides	K
Phazyme	K
Sulfasalazine (Azulfidine, Azo-Gantanol, Gantanol)	folic acid
Colchicine, Colbenemid	B12, A & potassium
Trifluoperazine (Stelazine)	B12
Cortisone (Tablets and Suspension, Orasone, Prednisone)	B6, D, C, zinc & potassium
Cathartic Agents (Epsom Salts)	K
(Atromid-S) Clofibrinate	K
Antacids (Maalox, Mylanta, Gelusil, Tums, Rolaids, etc.)	A & B (thiamin)

B.
IMPAIRMENT OF VITAMIN
UTILIZATION

*Vitamins
Depleted*

Coumarins (Dicumarol, Coumadin)	K
Pro-Banthine, Probital	K
Methotrexate	folic acid
Triamterene (Dyrenium)	folic acid
Pyrimethamine (Daraprim)	folic acid
Trimethoprim (Bactrim, Septra)	folic acid
Nitrofurantoin (Furadantin, Macrodantin)	folic acid
Phenylbutazone (Butazolidin)	folic acid
ASPIRIN	folic acid, C & B1 (thiamin)
Indomethacin (Indocin)	B1 (thiamin) & C
Bentyl with Phenobarb, Cantil with Phenobarb, Isordil with Phenobarb	K

C.
ENHANCED VITAMIN
ELIMINATION

*Vitamins
Depleted*

Aldactazide, Aldactone	potassium
Isoniazid (Inh, Nydrazid)	B6 (pyridoxine)
Hydralazine (Apresoline)	B6
Ser-Ap-Es (Serpasil, Apresoline and Esidrix)	B6
Penicillamine (Cuprimine)	B6
Chlorothiazide (Diuril, Diupres)	magnesium & potassium
Boric Acid	B2 (riboflavin)
Bronkotabs, Bronkolixer	K
Chardonna	K

II. Drugs with Multiple Mechanisms

Vitamins Depleted

Diethylstilbesterol (DES)	B6
Anticonvulsants	folic acid & D
Phenytoin (Dilantin)	folic acid & D
Barbiturates (Phenobarb, Seconal, Nembutal, Amytal, Butisol, Tuinal)	folic acid & D
Oral contraceptive steroids (Brevicon, Demulen, Enovid, Lo-Ovral, Norinyl, Ovral)	folic acid, C & B6
Alcohol	B1 (thiamin), folic acid & K
Betapar	B6, C, zinc & potassium

INDEX

Index